T0384732

Extrapolations: Demonstrations of Ericksonian Therapy

Ericksonian Monographs

Editor

Stephen R. Lankton, M.S.W.

Associate Editors

Ericksonian Monographs   Number 6

Extrapolations: Demonstrations of Ericksonian Therapy

Edited by Stephen R. Lankton
and Jeffrey K. Zeig

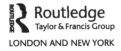

Routledge
Taylor & Francis Group

LONDON AND NEW YORK

First published 1989 by BRUNNER/MAZEL, INC.

Published 2014 by Routledge
2 Park Square, Milton Park, Abingdon, Oxfordshire OX14 4RN
52 Vanderbilt Avenue, New York, NY 10017

First issued in paperback 2014

Routledge is an imprint of the Taylor & Francis Group, an informa business

Library of Congress Cataloging-in-Publication Data

Extrapolations : demonstrations of Ericksonian therapy / edited by
Stephen R. Lankton and Jeffrey K. Zeig.
    p.   cm. — (Ericksonian monographs : no. 6)
Includes bibliographical references.
ISBN 978-0-87630-567-6 (hbk)
ISBN 978-1-13800-469-6 (pbk)
    1. Hypnotism—Therapeutic use. 2. Erickson, Milton H.
I. Lankton, Stephen R.   II. Zeig, Jeffrey K., 1947–
III. Series.
RC495.E97   1989
615.8'512--dc20

        89-37590
        CIP

Ericksonian Monographs

Ericksonian Monographs publishes only original manuscripts dealing with Ericksonian approaches to hypnosis, family therapy, and psychotherapy, including techniques, case studies, research and theory.

The *Monographs* will publish only those articles of highest quality that foster the growth and development of the Ericksonian approach and exemplify an original contribution to the fields of physical and mental health. In keeping with the purpose of the *Monographs*, articles should be prepared so that they are readable to a heterogeneous audience of professionals in psychology, medicine, social work, dentistry and related clinical fields.

Publication of the *Ericksonian Monographs* shall be on an irregular basis; no more than three times per year. The Monographs are a numbered, periodical publication. Dates of publication are determined by the quantity of high quality articles accepted by the Editorial Board and the Board of Directors of the Milton H. Erickson Foundation, Inc., rather than calendar dates.

Manuscripts should be *submitted in quintuplicate* (5 copies) with a 100–150-word abstract to Stephen R. Lankton, M.S.W., P.O. Box 958, Gulf Breeze, Florida 32562-0958. Manuscripts of length ranging from 15 to 100 typed double-spaced pages will be considered for publication. Submitted manuscripts cannot be returned to authors. Authors with telecommunication capability may presubmit one copy electronically at 2400, 1200 or 300 baud rate and the following communication parameters: 8 bit word size, No parity, 1 stop bit, x-on/x-off enabled, ASCII and xmodem transfer protocols are acceptable. Modem times are 7p.m. – 7a.m. CST on 904-932-3118.

Style and format of submitted manuscripts must adhere to instructions described in the *Publication Manual of the American Psychological Association* (3rd edition, 1983). The manuscripts will be returned for revision if reference citations, preparation of tables and figures, manuscript format, avoidance of sexist language, copyright permission for cited material, title page style, etc. do not conform to the *Manual*.

Copyright ownership must be transferred to the Milton H. Erickson Foundation, Inc., if your manuscript is accepted for publication. The Editor's acceptance letter will include a form explaining copyright release, ownership and privileges.

Indexing will include both name and keyword references. When submitting a paper, please list key words, key concepts and all names cited. These will be referenced across all papers so be judicious about choices, and do not include Dr. Erickson.

Reference citations should be scrutinized with special care to credit originality and avoid plagiarism. Referenced material should be carefully checked by the author prior to first submission of the manuscript.

Charts and photographs accompanying the manuscripts must be presented in camera-ready form.

Copy editing and galley proofs will be sent to the authors for revisions. Manuscripts must be submitted in clearly written, acceptable, scholarly English. Neither the Editor nor the Publisher is responsible for correcting errors of spelling and grammar: the manuscript, after acceptance, should be immediately ready for publication. Authors should understand there will be a charge passed on to them by the Publisher for revision of galleys.

Prescreening and review procedures for articles is outlined below. Priority is given to those articles which conform to the designated theme for the upcoming *Monographs*. All manuscripts will be prescreened, absented of the author's name, by the Editor or one member of the Editorial Board and one member of either the Continuing Medical Education Committee or the Board of Directors of the Milton H. Erickson Foundation, Inc.

Final acceptance of all articles is done at the discretion of the Board of Directors of the Milton H. Erickson Foundation, Inc. Their decisions will be made after acceptable prescreened articles have been reviewed and edited by a minimum of four persons: two Editorial Board members, one member of the CME Committee or the Board of Directors, and the Editor. Occasionally, reviewers selected by the Editor will assist in compiling feedback to authors.

Feedback for authors and manuscript revision will be handled by the Editor usually between one and two months after submission of the prepared manuscript. Additional inquiries are welcomed if addressed to the Editor.

Contents

Transcripts

Contributors

Joseph Barber, Ph.D., is Associate Clinical Professor of Psychiatry at UCLA. He is an assistant editor of *The American Journal of Clinical Hypnosis* and also serves as its book review editor. He is a fellow of both The Society for Clinical and Experimental Hypnosis and The American Society of Clinical Hypnosis, and is a diplomate of the American Board of Psychological Hypnosis. He received the Arthur Shapiro Award from the Society for Clinical and Experimental Hypnosis for the best book on hypnosis in 1983, for *Psychological Approaches to the Management of Pain* (co-edited with Cheri Adrian, Ph.D.). Barber has served as an invited member of the faculty of all the Erickson Congresses and Seminars since their inception in 1980.

Stephen G. Gilligan, Ph.D., is an international recognized authority on Ericksonian hypnotherapy who practices in San Diego. Gilligan has been an invited faculty member for all of the Congresses and Seminars organized by The Milton H. Erickson Foundation. He authored *Therapeutic Trances: The Cooperation Principle in Ericksonian Hypnotherapy*.

Stephen R. Lankton, M.S.W., is a professor of psychology at the University of West Florida, maintains a private practice in Gulf Breeze, Florida, and travels internationally to teach psychotherapy, hypnotherapy, and family therapy. Lankton is a fellow of the American Association of Marriage and Family Therapy. He has co-authored, with his wife Carol, *The Answer Within: A Clinical Framework of Ericksonian Hypnotherapy, Enchantment and Intervention in Family Therapy*, and *Tales of Enchantment: Goal-Oriented Metaphors for Adults and Children in Therapy*, and authored *Practical Magic: A Translation of Basic Neuro-Linguistic Programming into Clinical Psychotherapy*. Lankton has served as an invited faculty member at all of the Congresses and Seminars sponsored by The Milton H. Erickson Foundation. He co-edited *Developing Ericksonian Therapy* with Jeffrey Zeig and is the founding editor of the Ericksonian Monographs.

William Hudson O'Hanlon, M.S., maintains a private practice in Omaha, Nebraska, and travels internationally to teach Ericksonian and strategic methods. He was founding editor of the *The Milton H. Erickson Foundation Newsletter* and serves on the editorial board of the *Journal of Strategic and Systemic Therapies.* O'Hanlon co-authored *Shifting Contexts: The Generation of Effective Psychotherapy* (with James Wilk) and *In Search of Solutions: A New Direction in Psychotherapy* (with Michele Weiner-Davis), and authored *Taproots: Underlying Principles of Milton Erickson's Therapy and Hypnosis.* O'Hanlon has served as a primary faculty member for all of the Erickson Foundation Congresses and Seminars from 1981 to 1988.

Ernest L. Rossi, Ph.D., has been an invited faculty member to every Erickson Foundation Congress, Seminar, and Conference. As well as maintaining a private practice in Malibu, Rossi is a member of the editorial board of *The American Journal of Clinical Hypnosis* and is editor of *Psychological Perspectives: A Semi-Annual Review of Jungian Thought.* Best known for his collaborations with Milton Erickson, he has authored four books with Erickson, edited four volumes of Erickson's collected papers, and coedited three volumes of Erickson's early lectures. He authored *Dreams and the Growth of Personality: Expanding Awareness of Psychotherapy,* *The Psychobiology of Mind-Body Healing: New Concepts in Therapeutic Hypnosis,* and coauthored with David Cheek, *Mind-Body Therapy: Methods of Ideodynamic Healing in Hypnosis.* Rossi is a recipient of the Lifetime Achievement Award of The Milton H. Erickson Foundation.

Jeffrey K. Zeig, Ph.D., is Director of The Milton H. Erickson Foundation. He maintains an active private practice and regularly conducts teaching seminars on Ericksonian psychotherapy around the world. Zeig organized all of the Erickson Congresses and Seminars since 1980, including the landmark 1985 Evolution of Psychotherapy Conference. He serves on the editorial boards of two foreign and three American journals. Zeig edited or co-edited six books and co-edited with Stephen Lankton three Ericksonian monographs. He authored *Experiencing Erickson,* and a book about his work appears in Italian. His books are translated into seven languages.

Introduction

During the last 10 years, the mission of the Erickson Foundation has been to promote and advance the work of Milton H. Erickson, M.D. (1901–1980). This has been accomplished in a variety of forums: international congresses, conferences, seminars, regional workshops, the Milton H. Erickson Center for Hypnosis and Psychotherapy, the Evolution of Psychotherapy conferences, and publications, including the proceedings of the congresses, newsletters, and the Ericksonian Monographs.

Since 1981, at each of the annual congresses, conferences, and seminars, the foundation has asked invited faculty members to demonstrate their clinical work. The demonstrations are among the most popular events at the meetings and are videotaped for later study. October 29, 1989 marks the tenth anniversary of incorporation of the Milton H. Erickson Foundation, Inc. With this issue of the Ericksonian Monographs we offer an exciting complement to this anniversary.

For this volume, we solicited the six invited faculty of the tenth anniversary conference to select their favorite videotaped demonstration and comment upon it. The six faculty members are Joseph Barber, Ph.D., Stephen G. Gilligan, Ph.D., Stephen R. Lankton, M.S.W., William Hudson O'Hanlon, M.S., Ernest L. Rossi, Ph.D., and Jeffrey K. Zeig, Ph.D. For added perspective, we also asked each faculty member to comment on another faculty member's demonstration. The chapters in this volume were not subject to the normal editorial board review process but, rather, represent the complete and unabridged transcriptions for those demonstrations and the 12 commentaries.

Joseph Barber, "The First Session with Dr. B" (1984), with additional commentary by Stephen R. Lankton.

Barber conducts a first session with a client who presents a verbose treatment contract. During the session Barber demonstrates a remarkable skill-building rapport, making contact with the client and tracking the client, and being nonabrasive. His work with Dr. B. is rich with implications and awareness techniques. Indeed, his contact is so intense that the techniques and movement almost seem to flow from the client.

The commentary by Lankton illustrates additional considerations regarding the possible deliberate use of age regression and a diagnostic connection between other elements in the contract.

Stephen Gilligan, "Accessing Unconscious Processes" (1982), with additional commentary by Jeffrey K. Zeig.

Gilligan works with a client who had difficulty assessing the quality of her performance during test taking due to her apparent loss of contact with reality. His work with the client in trance uses embedded metaphors and anecdotes to illustrate the sequential acquisition of skills and to provide instructions for using natural rhythms of the body. Zeig comments on the session with thought-provoking ideas about Erickson's conceptions of induction, utilization, and responsiveness to indirect suggestion as they are so well-exhibited by Gilligan.

Stephen R. Lankton, "Motivating Action with Hypnotherapy for a Client with a History of Early Family Violence" (1988), with additional commentary by Joseph Barber.

Lankton's session is with a 42-year-old woman experiencing many self-critical thoughts and depression. She is an adult survivor of many types of early family violence. Lankton's interview style demonstrates his manner of curiosity and humor in these sensitive areas. The treatment techniques include a form of flooding for secure feelings (which previously created anxiety) followed by a metaphor to aid in identity-reassessment. The discussion by Barber points out that Lankton's diagnostic evaluation of the client reflects a broader understanding of the client than that presented with the symptom alone. While Barber is impressed by Lankton's "profound empathy with the client's phenomenology," he wonders about the necessity to embellish interventions with as much indirection and paradoxical intention as was demonstrated.

William Hudson O'Hanlon, "Solution-Oriented Hypnosis" (1988), with additional commentary by Ernest L. Rossi.

O'Hanlon explains his approach to "involuntary complaints" and demonstrates his work with a client who is anxious and having difficulty sleeping. O'Hanlon uses a sequential metaphor approach with illustrative anecdotes to help the client learn to relax. He also answers audience questions. In the commentary on his work, Rossi adds that the subject responded to suggestions for comfort and to the wide variety of stories used, but reminds us that Erickson was systematic in his use of such variety when he went "fishing" for diagnostic details in a first session.

Ernest L. Rossi, "Facilitating 'Creative Moments' in Hypnotherapy" (1985), with additional commentary by Stephen Gilligan.

Rossi explains many aspects of creative moments in his approach. He uses indirection to help clients become creative in areas where they previously stopped learning. With a series of four clients who had dreams, Rossi uses short interventions with questioning, channeling, and therapeutic binds to access resources. Gilligan reports on this demonstration by analyzing each of the four subjects in the session and focussing on Rossi's initial hypotheses. For instance, Rossi's emphasis on the "intrapsychic" uses of hypnosis to the apparent exclusion of the "interpersonal" aspects is of concern to Gilligan.

Jeffrey K. Zeig, "Using Metaphor and the Interspersal Technique" (1984), with additional commentary by William H. O'Hanlon.

Zeig's demonstration of utilization and hypnotherapy is with a client concerned about nuclear disaster, who is quite synesthetic and responsive to suggestion. His approach is one of embedded metaphor with an emphasis on developing the client's own inner strengths. O'Hanlon adds his two major concerns: that interspersed suggestions must be weighed carefully, and that genuineness must be present from the first handling of the client concern through the choice and delivery of real or imaginary metaphors in the session.

This issue presents, for the first time in print, these exemplary demonstrations of therapy and adds a valuable commentary by other experts. It reveals the influence of Milton H. Erickson's work on that of six professionals who have studied him carefully and extrapolated into their own work the essence they each took from his work. Companioned with the audio- and videotapes themselves (available from the Milton H. Erickson Foundation), this volume will serve as a valuable study guide for other serious investigators.

Stephen R. Lankton,
Gulf Breeze, FL
Jeffrey K. Zeig
Phoenix, AZ
May 1989

Extrapolations: Demonstrations of Ericksonian Therapy

The First Session with Dr. B

Joseph Barber, Ph.D.

Barber: What would you like to have happen in this meeting?

Dr. B: I have three aims. The first is to help me with the difficulty I have in doing hypnotherapy. I find that my thoughts do not flow as smoothly as they do when I do psychotherapy, and I feel I am blocking myself in some way which causes me to leave some notes on the table to prevent my forgetting things that might be my plan.

Related to this, I feel, let's say, that I am blocking myself somewhere in my appreciation of music; that is, when I am listening to a symphony I only hear the music here and now, and I somehow do not have the flow of what came before.

And if that is not enough work for you, I would like to improve the way I use my voice; that is, that very often I find myself—and I think that this is all related—putting pressure into my voice in order to be sure people will understand me. And this is very fatiguing to me, and it must be very unpleasant to the people who listen to me. And I am really only half aware of when I am doing it. But when I am doing it, I find it only rarely that I can stop myself from doing it. Once I've started on that pressuring the voice, I tend to stay with it.

Barber: Do you know how to stop it?

Dr. B: Yes.

Barber: Do you feel some pressured voice right now or does this feel pretty okay to you?

Dr. B: This feels pretty okay. I am tuned in to a certain frame and using my professional voice.

Barber: Is your voice as comfortable as you would like it to be, or is there some way that you would like it to be even more comfortable?

Dr. B: The voice could be slightly more comfortable.

Barber: Could you let yourself be a little more aware right now of what

---

Transcript of a demonstration given in Los Angeles, December 1984.

your voice is like, simply to see very specifically in what way you would like it to be a little more comfortable? What specifically?

Dr. B: When I speak with my professional voice, as I am doing now, there is a certain effort. I feel that this could very easily, I hope . . . ah . . . be totally natural without my making this effort to have a soft and pleasing voice, such as it is.

Barber: Well, would you be willing to speak effortlessly now, so I can hear what it would be like effortlessly? It doesn't have to be soft, or pleasing, or anything else. Just effortless would be interesting. What would that be like for you?

Dr. B: Well, we'll give it a try when the opportunity to say something comes along.

Barber: Okay. And how was that, just the, was that an effortless voice?

Dr. B: I think it was better; it was better already. Yes, slightly less effort in it.

Barber: What were you aware of in yourself that was different in creating that effortless voice as compared to what you call your professional voice?

Dr. B: Umm, forgetting about the effort to be professional.

Barber: Uh-huh. Well, I found it perfectly pleasing and perfectly easy to hear, so how about if we just try for a while with you speaking effortlessly. And if I find it unpleasing or hard to hear or something, I will tell you and you can put effort into it. Would that be all right?

Dr. B: All right. That's a good scheme.

Barber: So we have now cured one problem. What was the other one? Blocking yourself from appreciating some things, not only music, but I presume there may be other areas in your life that feel that inhibition.

Dr. B: In hearing, I am only aware of it with music, and I think that's why I can't carry a tune in a basket. But in hearing, I hear only the here and now, the immediate notes of the symphony, and I feel that there is some blocking in my observation of hypnotherapy patients. I do not feel that I am as in touch with them as I am with psychotherapy patients, where I have this feeling that it flows again. We come to the effortless nature of the thing, and I would like to accomplish that in hypnotherapy.

Barber: And how is your voice now, as we've been talking, is this your effortless voice, or is this effortful?

Dr. B: It seems rather effortless.

Barber: Ah . . . terrific. Okay. Can you tell me something more about what you know about this inhibition, this blocking of your own enjoyment, this blocking of your own appreciation, this blocking of your own contact with the world, both with respect to music and with your patients?

Dr. B: All right. Umm . . . my first memory . . . umm . . . relates to my father, who was an ear, nose and throat surgeon, piercing my ear drum. I must have been age 3 or 4, something like that. This relates also to the fact, I believe, that it has some significance that my father used hypnosis in his work as a surgeon, particularly with children. He was working at the children's hospital in Vienna, and he didn't like to use anesthetics. This is all ancient history. My father died 50 years ago, and he was operating from 1900 onward using hypnosis, and I was aware of the fact that he used hypnosis.

Barber: But he didn't use hypnosis when he was treating your ear?

Dr. B: I don't think so; I felt that piercing pain.

Barber: And how did you respond to that?

Dr. B: I screamed.

Barber: And how did your father respond to your scream?

Dr. B: It's funny that I do not remember my father in that incident at all, except as coming into the room. I remember two or three female figures in white, not really coats, but whatever nurses wear. I remember them as big heavy women, holding me. By the way, this was done at home, not at the hospital. I remember my father coming in, the piercing pain, and I scream. That's the end of the scene.

Barber: And is there a scene after that?

Dr. B: The scene immediately after that? Not now.

Barber: And where was your mother?

Dr. B: Very probably in the room, very probably one of the white clad figures.

Barber: And how was it that they were holding you? Were they holding you lovingly? Were they holding you distantly? Were they holding you with malice? How were they holding you?

Dr. B: I would say, "professionally" is the word that comes to mind.

Barber: So, they were holding you in order to get a job done. And how did that three-year-old feel about that, do you think, other than having a hurt ear? How otherwise did he feel about that?

Dr. B: Well, he screamed.

Barber: Did he scream in anger as well as hurt? Or was it only hurt?

Dr. B: A fury. Hurt and fury, I would say.

Barber: And you don't remember. But I just wonder, what that fury might have done . . . what form that fury might have taken in the moments following. The surgeon marches in, pierces the ear, marches out, and I wonder what form the fury of that young boy takes.

Dr. B: I have no idea.

Barber: And are you aware of any particular emotion now as you look down and say, "I have no idea"?

Dr. B: It just comes a little bit more, there's been some emotion since we've been talking about it, and when I start talking about fury. And . . . yes, there is a residual fear and emotion that comes back now that we are talking about it.

Barber: Is that all right with you?

Dr. B: Yes, so far, so good.

Barber: You tell me if we come to a limit about it.

Dr. B: I certainly will.

Barber: You weren't able to do it that day because you were very small, and there were four against one. But you can today.

Dr. B: That's good.

Barber: Okay. And what are you thinking right now?

Dr. B: I'm using the pattern on the carpet, I'm staring at it.

Barber: And as you stare at it, you can see it. Are you able to see it clearly?

Dr. B: Yes.

Barber: I wonder what comes into your mind if you just let yourself sort of playfully stare at the pattern on the carpet. I wonder if that reminds you of anything.

Dr. B: *(sigh)*

Barber: That's right.

Dr. B: It reminds me of some of these patterns that you see in the oriental designs. It reminds me of signs for the presence of atomic radiation . . . the signs for capsules . . . carpets in my childhood home . . . patterns in books relating to Jung.

Barber: Would you be willing to close your eyes,and let those patterns still be there in your mind's eye, those patterns you are looking at right now?

Dr. B: I'll see what I can do.

Barber: All right. Just get a good fix on those patterns. The reason I asked you to close your eyes is because I want you to have the opportunity to shift back and forth as it becomes appropriate between the patterns here and now and the patterns other places, other patterns in your mind. The pattern in this room is a pattern that can be very clear to you. Isn't it?

Dr. B: Uh-huh.

Barber: And are you able to see that pattern in your mind's eye?

Dr. B: Yes, I am.

Barber: Terrific. And this pattern also can remind you of other patterns from your memory, such as the patterns that describe the symbol for atomic radiation, and you can see that, or the pattern that advertises a particular brand of pill, you can see that?

Dr. B: Yes.

Barber: Or the patterns on the carpeting in your home as a child?

Dr. B: Yes.

Barber: Sometimes the patterns in your home would be more associated with one room, rather than another. I don't know what room you are most clearly associating to right now. Can you tell me?

Dr. B: Yes, I can. A very large entry hall that had patterned carpet and also a wood pattern on the wall that I am reminded of.

Barber: Wood pattern on the wall. And you look at the wood pattern with your eyes today, look at it very carefully, and just tell me if there is anything in particular that you notice about that wood pattern?

Dr. B: A wooden bunch of grapes.

Barber: A wooden bunch of grapes. When is the last time you saw that wooden pattern, except in your mind's eye?

Dr. B: Oh, other than in the photograph, I last saw that when I was 8 years old.

Barber: And where is this house?

Dr. B: In Vienna.

Barber: And you know the name of the street?

Dr. B: Yes, I do.

Barber: And what is that street name?

Dr. B: It's called the Gloriette Street.

Barber: Uh-huh. That's the English translation of the street name isn't it?

Dr. B: Gloriette Gasse, in German.

Barber: Uh-huh. And if we were to talk into that entrance hall, as you have done, suppose that you were to show me around inside your house. Where would be the first place you would like to show me?

Dr. B: Well, let's start with the entrance hall, where there is the patterned carpet which is blue and yellow, and where there is the natural-colored wood panelling. One of these panels has this grape pattern, which is really the only one that I remember now.

Barber: Are you and I the only people in this room? Are there others . . . any family members?

Dr. B: We can be the only ones in Vienna, I don't think we are the only ones in Los Angeles.

Barber: No, but in this room, in Vienna, is there anyone else walking back and forth through the room, or occupying the room?

Dr. B: Not now.

Barber: No. Okay. So just you and I are here at the moment. If someone else happens to walk into the room, will you let me know?

Dr. B: Of course.

Barber: And what else would you like to show me? I am interested in your house.

Dr. B: I like to eat and I like to sleep. And the dining room is immediately to the right, and I can describe it if it is of interest.

Barber: I wonder if we walk into the dining room, might there be a little something there to munch on?

Dr. B: There sure would.

Barber: So rather than describe having it, perhaps we could go in and have a small something.

Dr. B: Yes. All right. I like to do that.

Barber: And so what might we find here?

Dr. B: What comes to my mind is strawberry ice cream.

Barber: Strawberry ice cream. And who made this ice cream?

Dr. B: I believe the cook.

Barber: And what is cook's name.

Dr. B: Theresa.

Barber: Theresa. Does she make very good strawberry ice cream?

Dr. B: Very, very good strawberry ice cream.

Barber: What a lovely thing. And is it pleasing to you to experience this?

Dr. B: Yes, yes, there is some awkward feeling about it all, but it is a pleasing experience with an undertone of fear.

Barber: Yes, of course. And that's to be expected, isn't it? It would surprise you if it were otherwise, wouldn't it?

Dr. B: I have no expectations.

Barber: And yet, as a psychologist, you understand that very often when someone comes to you for something, that there is an amalgam of both excitement and perhaps hope, and perhaps delight, and also trepidation, and fear. That is a natural combination.

Dr. B: I think "trepidation" is a better word than "fear" for what I am experiencing.

Barber: And is your voice comfortable for you as we speak?

Dr. B: Comfortable, although a little awkward, at that last sentence, at this moment. Not that I feel that I am pushing it, but the discomfort that emotion can give to my voice.

Barber: Yes. What particular emotion is giving discomfort to your voice now?

Dr. B: Trepidation.

Barber: Uh-huh. Do you have any idea what we might find here that would be just a little bit frightening?

Dr. B: Yes, there would be a lot of bad scenes between my father and mother.

Barber: Is your father kind of an awesome character?

Dr. B: Very awesome, indeed.

Barber: If he were to come into this room right now, while you and I are in here nibbling on some strawberry ice cream, what might take place?

Dr. B: He would probably scream.

Barber: He would scream? What would he scream?

Dr. B: "What is this man doing here?"

Barber: Well, that would be pretty awkward for me.

Dr. B: Yes.

Barber: It would also be very rude on his part, wouldn't it?

Dr. B: Yes.

Barber: Is your father typically a rude man?

Dr. B. No. No. Only to members of the family. Not to strangers. Strangers would be protected.

Barber: I should think he would be a more gentle host to me?

Dr. B: He could be a very charming, and welcoming host, that's true.

Barber: So he might, on account of my being here, not scream at you?

Dr. B: He might scream at me and not at you.

Barber: But that would be also rude, wouldn't it?

Dr. B: It could be rude, yes.

Barber: I should think that it would be a social embarrassment for your father to scream at you in my presence. He doesn't know who I am.

Dr. B: Well, he was quite capable of that.

Barber: Just a moment ago, when your eyes opened, what was that like? And, now, what happens?

Dr. B: I opened my eyes because I was feeling a little bit dizzy, and so I thought opening my eyes would give me stability, which it does.

Barber: So, do you feel less dizzy now?

Dr. B: With the eyes open, yes.

Barber: And then when you close them, does the dizziness return?

Dr. B: Yes.

Barber: Would you be willing to experience it just long enough to see if I can help you resolve it without opening your eyes?

Dr. B: Of course.

Barber: If you need to stop the dizziness ahead of me, that's okay, but I'd like to see what we might do with it, because that's an interesting phenomenon, isn't it?

Dr. B: Right.

Barber: And are you feeling the dizziness now?

Dr. B: Yes, and it seems to be in the lower half of my body, rather than the usual dizziness that I might expect in my head.

Barber: So your head isn't dizzy; it's as if your body is dizzy?

Dr. B: The lower half of my body, yes.

Barber: About where does the dizziness begin? Where is the demarcation?

Dr. B: I would say at the hips, or just above the hips.

Barber: At the hips, or just above the hips, begins an area of dizziness throughout your lower body. And does it extend all the way to your ankles?

Dr. B: Yes.

Barber: And all the way into your feet?

Dr. B: To the big toe.

Barber: To the big toe. What a fascinating experience, and yet above your waist, you are not dizzy?

Dr. B: There's some tingling in the lower arms and hands.

Barber: Yes. And are you aware that one hand tends to tingle slightly more than the other?

Dr. B: Yes.

Barber: Would you be willing. . . . That's a pleasant tingling isn't it? It's not unpleasant is it?

Dr. B: It's indifferent.

Barber: Yes. So would you be willing to let that tingling increase if it does?

Dr. B: Yes.

Barber: That's fine. And when you decide that one hand is tingling significantly more than the other, will you tell me, and tell me which one? You don't have to worry. . . .

Dr. B: Yes. As you are talking the tingling is significantly stronger in the left.

Barber: In the left?

Dr. B: Yes. In the left hand and wrist, and almost disappeared from the right.

Barber: That's right. So the tingling that you experience in your left continues to increase even though it seems to virtually have disappeared in your right hand. And you haven't any need to explain that. You can just experience that for the moment. And I wonder if you would be willing to let that tingling increase almost to a sense of glowing, almost as if your hand can glow?

Dr. B: Yes.

Barber: And the tingling can extend, almost radiating through your wrist?

Dr. B: Yes.

Barber: And it might prevent you from fully appreciating the texture of your trousers beneath your fingers, and yet your right hand can pay as much attention to that cloth as you like. Do you notice that your left hand doesn't have the same appreciation of the material of your trousers?

Dr. B: It's different.

Barber: It is different, isn't it? And is the tingling below your waist still present?

Dr. B: No, that's pretty much gone.

Barber: Pretty much gone. That's very interesting. And so do you have no dizziness now at all?

Dr. B: Still in the thighs.

Barber: Still in the thighs. And does one thigh feel more dizzy than another?

Dr. B: Possibly the left.

Barber: Possibly the left. So the left hand tingles, the left thigh is more dizzy, and the right thigh seems to become less dizzy. Let me know when it virtually ends being dizzy altogether. And as you do that I want to suggest to you that you might feel another slightly disorienting experience. I am not certain, it might feel to you almost as if your body is leaning backward, as if you are floating in space, and as if your head is tipping backward. You know that isn't so, and yet you might occasionally have the feeling as if your head is tipping backward. And you might feel the need to pull it back. And I just want to suggest to you that you let it go and notice that you can't fall, because you are not floating in space. It may feel to you as if you are tipping back, as if there is nothing holding you out in space, but in fact you know there is, you know your feet are firmly grounded. You cannot fall, but you can be interested to experience that kind of peculiar floating, or dizziness, or instability. I'm not sure exactly what that is like, but you can tell me now what you are feeling.

Dr. B: As I move my head back, as I did before, I had the sensation that I might fall over backwards.

Barber: That's right. And so, as your head leans back sometimes involuntarily, you have to catch yourself so you don't fall. And yet, I want to suggest that you attend to the fact that right now you cannot fall. Right now the chair is holding you, you are not floating in space, and you cannot fall, and any impulse you have toward feeling as if you were falling is just an interesting illusion. An interesting illusion that you can experience as fully as you like, because I know that you have a particular interest in yourself and in your own mind. And this offers you one more opportunity yet to explore and to discover things that perhaps you haven't yet discovered. . . . And that as this continues I wonder if you are aware that some of the sensations in your throat have begun to change. And I am wondering if your throat feels more fullness or whether it feels more relaxed.

Dr. B: A bit dry, and a bit of dental anesthetic.

Barber: A little like an anesthetic. And is that comfortable or uncomfortable?

Dr. B: Indifferent.

Barber: It's indifferent. It's okay with you either way. All right. Well, I suppose that can just continue then. Nothing needs to happen that is so uncomfortable you cannot tolerate it. And yet there are such interesting things to experience, aren't there? And I wonder if you would be willing to let this kind of process continue to the extent that you actually experience an alteration in the way that your consciousness is operating. For instance, would it be all right for you to continue this experience by noticing a kind of catalepsy in the arm that tends to be dizzy? So in a moment then, I am going to lift your arm and I am going to leave it floating comfortably in the air, and I cannot predict whether it is going to float with stillness or whether the floating will be associated with interesting kinds of movements. I can't predict that. I don't really know. *(Barber lifts Dr. B's arm, which floats)* It doesn't really matter. But I would like you just to let it happen in whatever way seems most interesting and most natural to you, and I would like you to be willing to pretend for a moment that this is all happening without any effort at all on your part. I know that is only pretense and I'd like you to be willing to pretend, if you will, that for the next while, some things are going to happen that are totally outside effort. That for some reason they seem to happen with no effort at all on your part. It doesn't make them less interesting. It just makes them less effortful, if it were true, but it's only pretense. Is that all right with you?

Dr. B: Sure.

Barber: That's fine. And I'd like you just to let that floating continue, and if it turns out that your hand does continue to move in the direction that it has begun, that's all right. Or if it turns out that your hand begins moving in another direction, that's all right, too. How your hand moves is not important. What is important is the capacity of your mind to attend to the possibility of movement. How it is that you discover a kind of liberation from these various inhibitions and blocks . . . how you discover that is not what is important to me. What is important to me is that you have the capacity to allow that to happen when you feel properly prepared. . . . And I want to help you as best as I know how to feel prepared to just arrange for the subtlest alterations that can result in the greatest amount of liberation. *The smallest alteration that might result in the greatest liberation.*

And in a moment I am going to press down on your arm. Now when I do that, if I encounter some resistance to my pressure, that's all right, too. For instance, when you were a little boy, if you ever played with a wooden boat in the water, you know that if you press down on the boat it would just bounce back up. So you know, sometimes, resistance to pressure is perfectly natural. And yet everything can find its own level in its own way without any prior expectation or prediction. So, assuming that you can let this experience be the kind of experience you most want, I want to invite you just to let your mind float, no matter how fully grounded your body may feel, and just discover what it is that seems most compelling, of most interest to you. And as you do that you may find an annoying tendency for certain sounds or certain thoughts to pop up repeatedly. If so, just let that be, and continue anyway. And I would like you to feel free to let the development of this process continue, and I don't want to interrupt it. So suppose that you let the muscles of your voice, the muscles of breathing, the muscles of your larynx, of your jaw, of your lips and of your tongue . . . suppose you let those muscles become independently active for a while. So that without disturbing or interrupting or altering your experience in any way, your voice can just tell me what you are attending to right now?

Dr. B: Well, my attention is mixed: to that house in Vienna, and to your voice.

Barber: I haven't seen your room yet. I would be very interested if you would be willing to show it to me.

Dr. B: Well. . . .

Barber: How do we get there from the dining room?

Dr. B: Back out to the hall, and up the stairs, and to the top of the stairs.

Barber: Yes, tell me about this staircase. Is this the staircase that you ever get to play on?

Dr. B: Rarely . . . rarely.

Barber: When was the last time that you remember getting to play on this staircase?

Dr. B: I don't really remember a specific instance. Although I now remember very clearly the stairway and the carpet, and the wood and the wooden railing, and all those things.

Barber: The banister is very highly polished. Who polishes it?

Dr. B: Not my mother.

Barber: Not your mother. Who does polish it?

Dr. B: A maid.

Barber: And who is that?

Dr. B: No specific maid to that house.

Barber: Just a number of them. . . . Where is your mother right now as we climb the stairs?

Dr. B: In her bedroom. (sigh)

Barber: And is she often there?

Dr. B: Yes.

Barber: And do you ever visit her?

Dr. B: Yes.

Barber: And is that pleasant?

Dr. B: Yes.

Barber: What is she normally doing when you visit her in her bedroom? Is she resting?

Dr. B: Resting or putting on her makeup.

Barber: Uh-huh. And is your room down the hall from your mother's bedroom, or is it on another floor?

Dr. B: No, up. Up one floor.

Barber: Up one floor higher. This is a smaller staircase isn't it?

Dr. B: No, no. The bedrooms are on the same landing as that hall in the dining room.

Barber: I see. And where are we now?

Dr. B: Back in the hall.

Barber: And are we on the way to your bedroom?

Dr. B: We can be.

Barber: I would like that. Would that be all right with you?

Dr. B: That's fine. . . .

Barber: What do you see when you turn to your left in your mind's eye?

Dr. B: The top landing of that stairway.

Barber: And when you turn to the right?

Dr. B: Towards my bedroom.

Barber: Let's go over there, shall we?

Dr. B: All right.

Barber: It's an interesting smell in this house. How would you describe it?

Dr. B: Waxy.

Barber: Waxy. Is that what that is? You look as if something is delighting you right now.

Dr B: Mixture of wax smells and the wax, as opposed to your probable expectations.

Barber: And what's happening now?

Dr. B: I'm thinking of the scene when an outside doctor was brought into the house. Because as it turned out my brother had diphtheria, and this outside doctor, I remember very well, because he brought this most impressive microscope.

Barber: Could you tell me more about that?

Dr. B: I can tell you the doctor's name.

Barber: Uh-huh.

Dr. B: His name was Dr. Strauss.

Barber: Yes.

Dr. B: And I believe he had the binocular microscope. I believe that's the first time I had ever seen a binocular microscope.

Barber: Yes. And what became of your brother?

Dr. B: He grew up satisfactorily enough.

Barber: He survived the diphtheria?

Dr. B: He survived the diphtheria, yes.

Barber: And Dr. Strauss was impressive to you, but you didn't see him often.

Dr. B: No. I think he was brought because he had these special skills that went with the younger generation of doctors. He brought petri dishes and all kinds of wonderful things.

Barber: What are some of the other skills that you would have thought he would have as a younger generation of doctor? What are the kinds of things that you might have been able to expect from him, since he was of the younger generation?

Dr. B: I had no expectation. What comes to mind now, was that he could have been more of a children's doctor, but I happen to know he wasn't.

Barber: That's right. Since he was of the younger generation he had skills that were new, and so they wouldn't have been learned by the older generation? Is that what it seems?

Dr. B: That's right.

Barber: I wonder how some of those skills might be applied in a general sort of way, without any expectations, simply knowing that they are skills that are available, haven't yet been applied, haven't yet been appreciated, or realized, or benefited from. I wonder how they might be applied, and I wonder how at this moment, you might think of that.

Dr. B: Diagnosis, and then all of these things that have happened in medicine since then.

Barber: Yes. Is this an effortless experience at this moment, or are you pushing? Is that comfortable for you?

Dr. B: It's comfortable.

Barber: I'm finding myself wondering what the relationship might be between the blockage that you experience, the inhibition, the lack of contact in some ways you experience, and some of these very interesting and rich memories that you are having.

Dr. B: Well, I would think that there were a lot of things that were going on, as a matter of fact. And I know that there were a lot of things in my house to tune out on; and therefore maybe there was special interest in these wonderful things to tune in on.

Barber: So at a very early age, you began to learn how to avoid contact, to block awareness.

Dr. B: I would think I must have learned to tune out to a lot of spoken things.

Barber: Things that were too painful to hear?

Dr. B: Not painful, but unpleasant.

Barber: Unpleasant in a different sort of way, unseemly?

Dr. B: Unpleasant in the sense that the philosophy was "the truth is spoken here."

Barber: So they are unpleasant in the sense of being irritating?

Dr. B: Of being unnecessarily critical. In my opinion, it's not necessary to see everything, not necessary to speak about everything one sees.

Barber: You mentioned that when you are working with a patient in psychotherapy you are very observant. You feel like the process flows. You feel no particular blocks. But when you employ hypnosis you feel as if you have become blinded to certain things.

Dr. B: That I'm blocking myself, blocking myself both to what I see and observe. And I have to work, I have to put on a performance. I have to work hard, whereas my normal work flows.

Barber: Yes. Suppose that I am you in some way as a therapist. In what way might I be blinded right now? What occurs to you?

Dr. B: Well, if I were looking at myself sitting in this chair, I might want to ask what's behind the microscope and petri dishes, and what could be seen by looking into that microscope.

Barber: And what are you thinking right now?

Dr. B: I wonder how wise it is in this setting. I don't know.

Barber: Uh-huh. So, on the one hand you are curious, but there is that trepidation.

Dr. B: That's right.

Barber: Yes. And what's happening right now?

Dr. B: I'm nodding to the microscope.

Barber: And what is the microscope doing?

Dr. B: It's waiting.

Barber: It's waiting. It's waiting for you to look?

Dr. B: That's right.

Barber: Let's take a look. You don't have to tell me what you see, but let's just take a look.

Dr. B: Nice bacterial culture.

Barber: Can you identify the bacteria?

Dr. B: Diphtheria.

Barber: Diphtheria. And did Dr. Strauss let you look through the microscope to see it?

Dr. B: I'm sure he did.

Barber: A very privileged experience, wasn't it?

Dr. B: Yes.

Barber: And as you looked through the microscope at this bacterial culture, what ought I to ask you about that?

Dr. B: *(sigh)* What should those bacteria be doing to my brother?

Barber: Uh-huh? They are making him very ill, aren't they?

Dr. B: They sure are.

Barber: Yeah, and then you smile. I wonder what that feels like to you when you think of those bacteria invading you brother.

Dr. B: *(laughter)* It's not an unpleasant idea.

Barber: Is your brother older than you?

Dr. B: Older and smarter, bigger, faster, and stronger.

Barber: The bacteria kind of cut him down to size, don't they?

Dr. B: They do a beautiful job.

Barber: *(laughter)* Although Dr. Strauss was an eminent man, and in some ways a man that you admire, he also kind of got in the way, didn't he?

Dr. B: I have never thought of that.

Barber: Well, that's how it seems to me. I don't know . . .

Dr. B: Yes, I said I had never thought of that back then. I agree with you.

Barber: What would you like to say to those bacteria if you could look through the microscope again with both eyes? That's what's wonderful about this microscope: You don't have to limit yourself at all. I wonder what you would like to tell those little bugs.

Dr. B: Do a good job. *(laughter)*

Barber: And can you hear them talking back to you.

Dr. B: Yes, yes.

Barber: Do they feel pretty confident?

Dr. B: Yes, yes.

Barber: They know their work?

Dr. B: Very competent.

Barber: Very competent little bacteria. . . . If you could afford to in the context of your family, what would you like to tell Dr. Strauss?

Dr. B: Tell him my brother can take care of himself. *(laughter)*

Barber: He's very strong?

Dr. B: Yes!

Barber: If he's so smart, why isn't he well? Right?

Dr. B: Right.

Barber: And what would Dr. Strauss say?

Dr. B: It's good for you to catch diphtheria now rather than later.

Barber: Did you mean, it's good for you, or good for one?

Dr. B: Good for me.

Barber: Did you also catch it?

Dr. B: I disappointed him.

Barber: And did you disappoint your father?

Dr. B: I don't know.

Barber: It's hard to find out? Hard to know?

Dr. B: Uh-huh, he might go along with Dr. Strauss?

Barber: He might go along with Dr. Strauss. They are similar in many ways, aren't they?

Dr. B: They are doctors.

Barber: And they are trying to help your brother.

Dr. B: Uh-huh.

Barber: And you disappointed Dr. Strauss . . . What are you thinking right now?

Dr. B: I'm thinking about my father, and whether I disappointed him in not having diphtheria, if that was expected at that time. There might be a bit of confusion about that, that might have been about measles or something else at some other time.

Barber: Yeah.

Dr. B: And or whether I disappointed him in any other way.

Barber: Well, we need to begin thinking about how best to use this experience as it comes to an end, and I'm wondering if it would be interesting to you, to let yourself continue mulling over these interesting images of Dr. Strauss and his binocular microscope and his petri dishes. As you do that, keep entirely separate from that the fact that I would like to ask you to do something that may seem silly, but I mean it very seriously, which is I would like you, on the one hand, to pretend that you see all that needs to be seen by a mortal human when you are working with your patients hypnotically, and to assume that you are always missing something, just as any mortal human would. Does that dichotomy make sense to you in a way that you can pretend both of those, equally fervently, at the same time?

Dr. B: (nods his head)

Barber: Terrific. And is there anything else in particular that you would like to tell me, or you would like me to say to you, before we end this experience today?

Dr. B: Uh-huh, just some suggestions about trance being more easily available to me.

Barber: My understanding of you, however briefly developed, is that you have a great capacity for developing trance, and that you limit yourself quite reasonably as a way of protecting yourself from these unknowns that give you such trepidation. And I don't know how to suggest to you that you ought not to feel trepidatious, and I don't know how to suggest that you simply ignore that. There are unknowns. I think you are taking care of yourself pretty well.

Now, you are a cautious man in some ways, and so you may be overcautious with yourself about this. You may be underestimating a lot of your own capacity about this, about how you can take care of yourself in less constricting ways. Those things occur to me to say to you. I will be very interested, however, if I have the opportunity to discover, in the not too distant future, some things that you began to learn from now. For instance, I wouldn't be surprised if you begin remembering certain features of your dreams, and having some kind of understanding as a result of that. Nor would I be surprised to find out in some way being a hypnotherapist enables you to feel differently about your work. I would be interested to know that when the time comes. Would that be all right with you?

Dr. B: Good.

Barber: Terrific. Well, what I would like you to do then, is to just let yourself reflect for a moment then, about what we have done, and what we have experienced, and to let your mind flow, and to let your mind reorient to the fact that in just a moment we are going to go back out into the world of Los Angeles, and that you will want to have the things arranged in your own mind the way that is most comfortable for you. And then, when you feel ready, you might just take a refreshing, energizing breath and find yourself sitting with your eyes open, and vaguely curious about what it is that you might look forward to.

(Pause)

Barber: And how are you feeling right now?

Dr. B: Pleasant. Soft.

Barber: Terrific. And how is your voice right now?

Dr. B: Pleasant and soft.

Barber: Okay, thank you.

Dr. B: Thank you.

Commentary

Joseph Barber, Ph.D.

I especially appreciated the fluency with which Dr. B was able to move from his initial presentation of his problem ("blocking" in his own hypnotherapeutic work, "blocking" in appreciation of music, and "effortful" use of his voice) to his awareness of long-unexpressed pain and fear.

In my work with Dr. B, I tried to orient him to awareness of his present experience, to better avoid intellectualizing about his experience. His communications were especially rich in meaning, and much future work could be based on this conversation alone.

Initially, of course, I listened to Dr. B to understand what he wanted. His presentation was essentially intellectual, and my conjecture was that he wanted something more than he was able to say at that time. My first intervention was to ask him to speak effortlessly (since one of his presenting problems was speaking effortfully). There were three reasons: 1) to discover if it was possible (and, if so, to demonstrate that it was); 2) to discover what, if anything, might be associated with this; and 3) to find a point from which we could attend to his present experience.

The second intervention was to express my curiosity about what other things (besides the appreciation of music) might be inhibited and to ask him to tell me more about his inhibition, implying that the inhibition was related to contact with the world. Dr. B's response to my inquiry was to begin telling me a childhood memory of fear and pain.

My focus then was to maintain what Erv Polster (1983) calls "tight sequentiality" with Dr. B—to follow closely, moment by moment in his experience. I wanted to help him to become absorbed in his memories and to make them as emotionally and sensorally present (rather than merely intellectual) as possible. I spoke to him as if the memories were happening in the present. I was suggesting a form of age regression, and continued in this mode throughout the remainder of the conversation.

Finally, I offered Dr. B a variety of suggestions intended to normalize his day-to-day experience, and to create a more self-accepting attitude.

Reference

Polster, E. (1988). *Every person's life is worth a novel*. New York: Norton.

Commentary

Stephen R. Lankton, M.S.W.

Barber's first session with Dr. B is a superb example of many of the relationship and technical factors that ought to occur in a first session. The tasks of a first session include establishing rapport, liking the client, gathering data, understanding the request for therapy, contracting, instilling hope, outlining a direction for progress, and making what progress one can. This is a great first session, and readers should know that it needs to be listened to, instead of merely read, to be fully appreciated.

What I like best about this session is the manner in which Barber seems to accomplish the tasks of an initial interview with apparently little effort. His style is replete with directed implications, awareness, and clarity of thought and articulation. But none of the techniques get in the way of his contact with the client.

I particularly like the way he respectfully relates the presentation of a potentially "shallow" contract to the broader life issues of the client. Specifically, the client said that he felt that he was "blocking myself somewhere in my appreciation of music; that is, when I am listening to a symphony." However, Barber soon inquires, "Can you tell me something more about what you know about this inhibition, this blocking of your own enjoyment, this blocking of your own appreciation, this blocking of your own contact with the world both with respect to music and with your patients?"

I mentioned that Barber's speech is rich with implication, nuance and binds. Let us dissect a stylistic technique used by Barber. He says to the client, "So how about if we just try for a while with you speaking effortlessly. And if I find it unpleasing or hard to hear or something, I will tell you and you can put effort into it." The client agrees. The delivery of this request is natural and conversational. So much so that a viewer might be reluctant to call this a "technique." I doubt that Barber would call it a technique. And this is exactly as it should be. The technique and the therapist are one. Barber illustrates and models a type of sanity that might be called "standing behind your words."

Throughout the session he relies upon "gestalt awareness techniques," and the ensuing hypnotic aspects of the relationship are due primarily to those methods; examples abound in Barber's transcript. One of the more important moments for any of us in therapy are those times when clients give little information. On one occasion, Barber inquires, focussing awareness, "I wonder what form the fury of that young boy takes." To this the client replies, "I have no idea." Barber then asks, "And are you aware of any particular emotion now as you look down and say, 'I have no idea'?" The client answers that there is some fear, and Barber follows with the question, "Is that all right with you?" Thus, moving smoothly to fertile information but also doing something else of importance.

Behind that question, as well as others, we find a position of the so-called new epistemology that has often been credited to Erickson's work. It is a posture of putting one foot in the client's world and leaving one foot in your own, and treating the client as an individual. I am heartened by this posture. Barber does not presume to know a great deal from this answer from the client about his problem. Instead, he inquires about the client's experience and its meaning at every step of the session. Far too often therapists, with little information, begin to mold clients into their favored theories. I suspect this is done by therapists to help themselves feel secure with the role of helper. Yet, they do not truly help when this is done. Barber, however, demonstrates the security of a true helper by entering into a dialogue with his client and moving in small steps—always keeping the integrity of the client's experience in the foreground. There is, therefore, no need to "do" for the client. Barber leads the client to "do" for himself.

Thinking on what I would have done differently, one major fact comes to my attention. This is a *first* session with a client who might not have sought psychotherapy for the presented concerns. The offering from the client was so vague (musical awareness) it might be too much to expect more movement. Since a first session is all we get in this transcript, it would be inappropriate to judge what sort of treatment procedure could have been used in place of that which occurred.

I wondered about the voice tone and vocabulary used by the client throughout. By both tone and words the client seemed intellectually distant, well educated, and mature. In many instances, Barber talked with the client as if an age regression were presupposed, yet the client maintained an intellect more representative of an adult. Perhaps it was a regression in age to a precocious child. I recall that the client was concerned with putting pressure in his speech so people would understand him, and I wonder if a precocious child would be motivated to pressure his speech.

In light of that development, I would have questioned the desire for an age-regression/reliving-gestalt. If such a regression or reliving was desired, a departure from the style of communication presented could have included helpful suggestions for age regression beyond the presuppositions used. This might have resulted in a more interesting set of data than that which was elicited through the adult intellect of the client. Further, the client may have been able to unearth a younger part of himself who did not want or need to pressure his speaking in an attempt to get others to understand. A more apparent hypnotic experience, however, would have needed to follow a successful attempt to protect the client from pain. He has, after all, told us that his father did a therapeutic procedure on him in the presence of others but with little regard for his comfort or need for anesthesia. Still, one must consider the setting, the contract, and the client's motivation. Perhaps, in this demonstration setting, the style of conversation used was more effective, in that it provided a degree of protection from what otherwise might have been *too* revealing in a congruent therapeutic age-regression.

Accessing Unconscious Processes

Stephen G. Gilligan, Ph.D.

Gilligan: You've asked to come up here and volunteer for some explorations on a particular issue that you have in mind. Would you mind briefly describing that to the others?

Connie: Yes. I take comprehensive exams in September, and I'm a very good student, but I tend not to have any sense of knowing what I know; and I have to integrate 3 years worth of material. And when I take exams ordinarily, I go into trance, so I don't remember later what I've written or have any sense of really knowing that information when I'm not in trance.

Gilligan: Now, you do well on your exams in the trance?

Connie: Yes.

Gilligan: Now, what do you think concerns you then about not doing well, or apprehension that you may not do well, on the coming test if you went into a trance?

Connie: Because this requires a great deal of integration. To study for one exam means to memorize maybe 80 pages. That's not a difficult task. . .

Gilligan: Oh, no. I'm sure everybody in the audience agrees with you. *(laughter)*

Connie: Over time, over time, but 3 years worth of material, I don't trust myself to be able to integrate that much. And the kind of questions they ask are questions that will cover many courses.

Gilligan: So you think you would like to forego a trance on exam day?

Connie: No, no. I think I would like to go into trance when I start studying in June and just stay in trance until exam. *(laughter)*

Gilligan: You don't live in California, do you?

Connie: No.

Transcript of a demonstration given in Dallas, December 1982.

Gilligan: I think I know where that's legal. *(laughter)* Okay. Now you've had a lot of previous trance experience.

Connie: Uh-huh.

Gilligan: Any with me?

Connie: I did a workshop with you in Chicago, but I didn't work with you individually.

Gilligan: Do you remember the group? Did you experience a trance as a member of that group? What position were you in at that time?

Connie: I was a student.

Gilligan: And your body position?

Connie: Oh, that position. *(she adjusts her posture)*

Gilligan: Okay, now what I would like to do, I think, is demonstrate for the others and offer for you some communication regarding how dissociational processes can be used in various ways. Now, if I am correct in hearing you and talking with you earlier, one of the things that you would like to do is to be able to experience dissociation, and yet have some assurance that the integration is going on—the integration will be able to manifest itself on test day. Now.

Connie: In fact, as I'm studying, so I would have some secure sense that I was utilizing the time well.

Gilligan: And right now you experience dissociation without much conscious awareness about what happens. Is that par for the course in trance experiences for you?

Connie: What do you mean?

Gilligan: Is that what typically happens in all situations when you develop a trance?

Connie: No, it would depend on how deep the trance was.

Gilligan: Okay. Now, do you experience hand movement in trance?

Connie: Uh-huh. [Yes]

Gilligan: And you have a "yes" finger? *(pause; the index finger lifts up)*
(After a lull, there's laughter)

Gilligan: Now that goes to show you—we're both sitting here in front of a large audience, right now. And you can look at me *here* and *hear* me *here*; recognize for *now* that out *there* are them; recognize also that you needn't hear *there*; involved perhaps now, however, it is the case. *(pause; looks at hands again)* And a "no" finger? It is as if you have experienced . . . You've got the ability consciously to respond. You've also got the ability to *unconsciously respond* . . . and you can develop the awareness to recognize the difference between the two. Now a moment ago, I asked about the "yes" finger, and there are two types of lifting: A right finger begins to jerk, just like the hand, *up*. And also then, effortful voluntary movement. And both can really complement the other, as long as they don't compete. Now, how do you feel right now?

(Connie develops eye fixation on her hand, with body catalepsy)

Connie: Relaxed.

Gilligan: Relaxed. And what are you aware of developing in visual awareness?

Connie: I'm aware of your face . . . and the light . . . and my eyes to my right primarily.

Gilligan: And has my face begun to change *yet*?

Connie: No.

Gilligan: Has the feeling in your hands begun to change *yet*?

Connie: Yes, there is a tingling in my right hand.

Gilligan: A tingling in your *right* hand? And has the feeling in your feet begun to change yet?

Connie: They're tingling.

Gilligan: Do you enjoy that tingling?

Connie: Sure.

Gilligan: Has the feeling in your eyelids begun to change yet?

Connie: No.

Gilligan: Has the feeling in your chest begun to change yet?

Connie: Heavy.

Gilligan: And your visual awareness?

(Connie continues unblinking eye fixation, suggesting tunnel vision)

Gilligan: And your left hand? . . . Now, one of the suggestions that I would like to offer is that you have a variety of different experiences of trance already under your belt. One of the nice things that you can do is be able to *reorganize* certain hypnotic responses so they occur in a complementary fashion. Whether it's the feet, and the sensation may be right and left foot *changing;* or whether it's the hands, and feeling right and left hands *changing;* or whether it's my face, and the lighting on my face *changing,* the fact of the matter still remains: You really *can* continue to wonder, to question. You really *can* continue to recognize that it's important, to *hold out* just a little bit, and it's important also to wait [weight], wait [weight], wait on the one hand. And on the other hand to recognize that sense of urgency is sometimes a product of the moment, and all moments are transitory. I know, for example, that in the past week, past month, past year for that matter, I've been completing my doctoral dissertation. I know that in the last month I sat rather *intensely* . . . in my office . . . at my word processor . . . and typed over and over and over and over and over again. And my hands began to feel that they were operating *independently.* I didn't have to think, "Where's the i on the keyboard?" I didn't have to think, "Where's the return on the keyboard?" I didn't have to think, "Where's the delete?" In an automatic way, utilize those different elements as keys to translate thoughts. What a nice thing about modern technology, word processors, that you can really *reorganize* on the spot. I know, for example, that in writing my doctoral dissertation, I wrote.

(Connie begins to close eyes)

Gilligan: You shouldn't go *too* quickly now, Connie. That's a tendency that should be avoided. You really don't have to leave. You can let the situation *alter* of its own accord. Or you can use the word processor. You establish different documents on different records. I know that in my 150-page dissertation there are many different documents. Fifteen pages of references, figures, tables, introduction, experiment 1, experiment 2, 3, 4, 5, 6, and general discussion. Well, it came time to print it out for acceptable copy. I had to use document link on the word processor. Never could do that on the typewriter. *(pause)* One of the wonderful things that you can learn is to be able to *respond selectively.* Now whether it is that hand that's operating *independently,* or whether it's your eyelids blinking *up* and *down* independently. *Down* again— up—*down*—independently—up—*down,* independently. Or the feet *tingling.* You *can* recognize what is that metaphor, and recognize a symbolic alteration. Sometimes very fitting. And people have idiomatic phrases. "If the shoe fits, wear it." Well, what happens if the shoe does not fit? And you can be able to outfit yourself . . . with clothing proper not only for mundane expression, not only for transitory expression, but a symbolic expression of *reorganization* in a manner that is appropriate for you as an individual.

And so you can let yourself become aware of visual realities, and you recognize also that a kinesthetic development, a *somatic* development can also be par for the course. You can be able to really enjoy . . . a birdie, an eagle. And recognize that you can score . . . soar . . . score with the best of them. And you can do that in so many different ways, Connie. I know, for example, yesterday Jeff Zeig telling me of his newly acquired hobby of gliding—of learning how to fly glider planes. And he described to me how exhilarating it was just to be able to go along all by himself. And he started out with a lot of investment, with a lot of guidance, supervision. But soon Jeff's at the control all by himself. And he invited me to *learn about gliding.* I didn't know if it was going to be appropriate. I certainly could *imagine* being able to glide from a perspective up on high and be able to look down and see all those different patterns and all different combinations and connections of urban and rural . . . a patchwork of farming, of smoke stacks and playing fields, of little boys and girls playing ball, of men and women going to work, and the ability of really being able to enjoy the *perspective* gained from hang gliding. As I already told Jeff, "I don't know. I certainly will *think about it.*" And that brought a lot of conscious orientation. . . . But there's some fear involved; some anxiety involved.

Now, I know another experience, in growing up, my brother and I were very close. Everywhere my brother went, I went, dressed in the same clothes—red cardigan sweaters—going to Mass every Sunday. My brother is several years older. And all the time, the term "the boys" was used to refer to him and me. And growing resentment, a growing recognition of the need for awareness between the two. My brother and I turned into fierce competitive individuals who wouldn't give each other the time of day. I had to *learn* to *separate* with an *awareness* so that I could engage in tasks that were interesting for me, he and his. We both stopped wearing red cardigan sweaters. It wasn't until I learned about unconscious response, that I began to recognize how many different needs for autonomy and different expressions of autonomy one can have. Oh, a nice *uplift* that one can be able to develop from psychological experience of recognizing reorganization of different, sidetracks of different, symbolic instances of different manners of being able to express differing, opportunities for difference, experiences of dissociational intelligent autonomy. And whether *it is* finger twitch, *lift up*, hand *up*, press down *(hand begins to levitate)*, whether *it is* memory from the past, childhood memory. Whether it is tingling, alteration, auditory perception. Whether *it is* onset shortly of dream as soon as hand *lifts*, only as soon as you recognize own way, own time. And you really can recognize what is a metaphor.

And if you live in California, you recognize contrast: mountains and coasts. And going *up* the coast you can recognize how fog can obscure a view, a very beautiful contrast. Growing up in San Francisco, it's hard sometimes to see only a block away. *You can't see beyond that block.* I took my initial education in San Francisco and then Santa Cruz. Both very foggy and both really obscuring vision beyond one block. And luckily, I moved to Palo Alto . . . *take a trip.* Move a distance away, still close enough to the old learning institutions. But one thing very nice about Palo Alto . . . never foggy. You can see for a long way, and it's always nice to know that in any environment, *there's always more beyond the block.* And your unconscious really can demonstrate, Connie. And recognize that you really can let yourself develop that depth of trance, really can let yourself recognize that there can be concerns, there can be doubts, there can be worries, should be, will be, always will be, but along with that *the unconscious response*—perhaps imperceptible at first *(hand jerks up)* . . . that's right, a little bit more, Connie, enveloping *all in good time.* As you can operate in *good* time. You really can have a *good* time. And recognize those manifestations, different realities, can, should occur, with a mixture of *different life experiences*. I know that at training martial arts students I learned the joy of pain and pleasure. I learned the satisfaction derived from frustration and completion. And I learned the necessity of *contact* and *withdrawal*. I learned the importance of *holding on, letting go*. And at a martial arts studio, a casual observer often asked after an intense test, *"How can you possibly test so hard and not really have unpleasant feelings about it?* Are you throwing kicks here, you throwing punches there? You're integrating everything seemingly. Different combinations—punches and kicks, right hand and left hand, right leg, left leg. And how do you do that?" *(pause)* I know that in training at the martial arts students that you drill them in ways they can enjoy. For example, you can number a hand—left hand 1, right hand 2, left foot 3, right foot 4—and you have them jog in place, dance around in place, and listen to the instructors call out the numbers: 1 and the left hand there has movement; 2, right hand; 1,2, a combination of different movements; 1,2,3, left hand, right hand, left foot; 4,2,1, right foot, right hand, left hand; 1,3,4, left hand, left foot, right foot; 1,3,4: *and the middle third, the center of the integration* also predominant, but always keep them running comfortably. You work up a sweat. You should. And you *discover different combinations*. They can be generated from different formal forms that you have learned. And so rather than going through Pinon 1, Pinon 2, Pinon 3, Pinon 4, Pinon 5, and going through all the different forms, you put them together in different combinations. And you learn in martial arts the importance of combinations in formal forms and placing 24 movements together. And their predicted sequence and taking them apart again. Every student will come in and look and want to throw a jump . . . spin . . . hook . . . reverse kick, right off the bat. Especially the youngsters who come in, adolescents, will want to do exactly what the black belt is doing, will want to know: How do I throw a jump, double spin, hook kick? And they demonstrate the fact that if they throw that too fast, too quickly, they are going to land right on their butt. And so you stress the importance of *stretching*—the importance of being able to take a little time—not only before a test, but before each workout. And really let yourself limber up physically, limber up emotionally, limber up physically. Are you ready to let your muscles stretch? Because in letting those muscles stretch, what your body is learning to do is to discriminate different muscle groups . . . Individuals first come in and throw a punch with the entire body—muscles bunch up and tense. Mental awareness is very focused and violent. They really have little power and are off balance. You learn with stretching. You learn through forms. You learn through combinations, 1, 3, 2, and continue on, exploring all the different permutations: 1, 1, 2, 1, 3, 4, 1, 1, 1, 1, 1, 1, 1, 1, one, won. And it really is nice to know that "won" can be in the past tense, and you really can know it can be a *present* in the past tense, and know that which was *then* a present, can become *now again* in the future—an utter actuality. And whether you wear white, yellow, green, blue, purple, brown, black, you really can recognize—those different combinations of training as opportunities to discriminate, to strengthen associations, and gain flexibility. And sometimes individuals express surprise when they find out I have a black belt. They say you don't look overly muscular. I really have to tell them that *you don't have to overpower it. You learn to operate in accord with internal rhythm.* You learn to operate in accord with flexibility. And you let those violent, muscle-bound people lunge right by. Let *all* those anxieties drift right on by. I recognize that 1, one, won, 1 . . . is a result of repetitive and yet flexible and intelligent investigation. And your unconscious really can operate in accord with the present needs, and present understanding. I know, for example, that working with one individual colleague at Stanford University, a colleague approached me, asked me if I though that lucid dreaming was a psychological possibility available to anyone. I said I didn't know. It sounded like an interesting research project, and I consented to help him out devising methodology for a lucid dreaming. And so the contemplation of the question: *How do you develop a lucid dreaming state?* It was something that had to be thought over. Food for thought, not only in dreams; food for thought when I was studying other methodologies as well. And I worked with the experimental subjects and trained them to develop a very deep trance, and operate in a very deep trance . . . and *let the unconscious do the learning (Connie moves head slightly)* make the adjustment, head *down, up, over to areas of learning that were going to be important.* And I gave those individuals suggestions so they could *practice lucid dreaming.* And they had at least six dreams every night. I didn't know which one, which dream in the first week was going to be devoted to lucid dreaming. And how can you have a lucid dream and forget that it was lucid? And over the weeks, a development of higher frequencies of lucidity, of awareness of dissociational processes, of awareness of the function of dreams, of the awareness of the ability of the unconscious to integrate, to develop, to explore, to combine learnings in various experiential ways appropriate to the needs of the entire self. *You can feel it. You can feel it. You can feel it. (long pause)* And a tiny seed. And yet the beauty of a rose, of a bud, and the patience . . . of letting that bud . . . *open up* at the appropriate time. And now, that the enjoyment of any rose is occasionally tempered by a thorn. What else is new?

And so my colleague at Stanford mapped out the frequency of reported lucid dreams in a number of subjects and found that all his subjects could *learn lucid awareness of dissociational processes.* And dreaming really is only one way the unconscious *can* operate. And you can be able to occupy your time in gardening; you can occupy your time learning martial arts; you can occupy your time at a word processor; you can occupy your time running around the track; you *could* operate and occupy your time worrying, but *always, always, always* you can let remain across all of that transitory reality, the recognition of the *autonomy of the unconscious.* The *security* and *trust.*

I know, for example, that an individual, a friend of mine, was studying for a premedical exam. I was very very concerned that she was going to be overwhelmed by the anxiety, because in one day of MCATs she was going to have to go through biology, chemistry, literature, reading comprehension, physics, and she didn't know how she was going to be able to do it all. I told her, "I don't know either exactly how *you'll do it.*" But I do know your unconscious can *get to work.* And your unconscious can . . . *take care of it.* And she worried and worried and studied and worried and studied and worried, and got up her hopes and studied some more, and got discouraged and studied some more. Had a snack and went for a walk, studied some more, worried and took pleasure in a TV show, worried, studied, studied, and enjoyed relaxation trance, deep trance, worried a little bit less, but still some. And the *right* to worry, to be *left* with *a middle third of security* all the while, no matter which side of the issue you do explore. And recognition in doing so, that *always, always, always* the unconscious has a lot more capacity than a 56K word processor. And has a lot more functions than simple deletion, or return that you can press on a typewriter: *Return, Return, Return.* Until you hear that chatter in a typewriter; it can be very annoying and distracting. I know, for example, that I used to write on a typewriter, and didn't think I could think without all the chattering of the keys. I didn't realize how useful a word processor can be, and how much more useful it was to be able to see my results on the screen in front of me. And so I told my friend studying for her MCATs that her unconscious could get to work. And she found herself thinking back to childhood experiences, very pleasurable, very secure experiences. And she had some very friendly dragons. Other people heard about that and said, "Dragons friendly?" And her dragons were very friendly. Her "Prince Charming." And she could use those dragons to slay all her other obstacles, and she was very delighted to recognize that those dragons could sit on her shoulder and she'd still have all of the burden on her shoulders, and with the dragon on her shoulder there would be no room left for other associations. That is, you don't want to get *too close* to a dragon. *(pause)*

Now when a kitchen gets too hot, you know what you need to do. And so you can recognize, you can let your unconscious *cool things.* Everybody does have their own style, Connie. And so I don't know exactly how it will happen for you. I know, for example, one day a group of black belts were standing around, and I began to talk about how I control pain by experiencing it as heat and allowing it to emanate out and escape from my fingers and toes; and that is a way to control pain. And Rodney, a 3rd degree black belt, said "No, whenever it gets painful for me, I just think of my girlfriend." He said, "I let myself experience pleasure of being with my girlfriend, and then that pain is enjoyable tingling of a degree that I can't share with you here." And Chris, a 2nd degree black belt, said that his body got completely numb and he felt very detached. And you really can learn combinations appropriate for the situation. Based with one situation, a 1, 1, 1, 2, 4, meta 4; 2 . . . 4 . . . 3, meta 4; 4, meta 4; 5 . . . symbolic alteration; 6 . . . flexible combinations; 7 . . . a lucky day; 8 . . . the experience of a good meal, and the satisfaction of knowing that you can nourish yourself more than once a day; 9 . . .10 . . .10 . . . really can attend to unconscious needs; 11 . . . a repetition that provides a new meaning. . .

And Gregory Bateson used to point one plus one is not always two—sometimes three; and he would joke that he would put a wife and a husband together, one plus one sometimes you got three. And you talk about putting two patterns against each other, and you'd get a third pattern. And I pointed out that you can put one beside another one, and *get eleven.* And *whoever heard of a* psychological Baker's dozen anyway? Well, you can skip some that are not important, and continue on in that progression. And you can let the unconscious take care of things. And I like to take every night a substitute for the prayers I used to say when I was a youngster. I thank my unconscious in drifting off, and I acknowledge the unconscious is a smart cookie, and I begin to orient to a different state. But no matter what state that you orient to—Massachusetts, Arizona, Texas, California—you really can recognize the unconscious as a bonafide citizen of the United States of Consciousness. What a nice thing to know . . . that you can enjoy that citizenship and let your vote *count* on election day and feel the satisfaction of bringing home a *winner.*

And so in a moment, Connie, I'm going to begin to count backwards from ten to one, as I do you can reorient from trance. Bring back only that which is appropriate to bring back. 10 . . .9 . . .8 . . .7 . . .6 . . . 5 . . .4 . . .3 . . .2 . . . *(eyes open)* And you fill in the rest!

Connie: Uh-huh.

Gilligan: And you recognize what its present tense is . . . And what its future tense will be . . . People say that there is no negation . . . that can be demonstrated unconsciously. Would you subscribe to such a hypothesis?

Connie: Uh-huh.

Gilligan: So would I, but with one exception. *You can reject anything. (long pause)* Now how does your right hand feel?

Connie: Fine.

Gilligan: Are you surprised?

Connie: No.

Gilligan: Take a deep breath. *(long pause)* And how are you feeling?

Connie: Fine.

Gilligan: Take your time in reorienting back fully. I know this can be an unusual situation here. You don't have to force yourself to orient back out into the group at large until you feel appropriate about doing so. Okay? *(Connie nods head)* And I want to thank you very much.

(Turns to audience)

Gilligan: I'm willing to open the floor in a Moses-like fashion to any comments or questions from the "peanut gallery," if you don't mind. Any questions? I think we have time, for a couple of minutes, if there are any? If you do, you'll have to come up to the microphone.

Gilligan: *(to Connie):* Feel free not to answer if you don't want to.

Member of the audience: What was the purpose of the hand motions that you did, and were you aware of hand motions, and what happened when you noticed them?

Gilligan: *(to Connie):* Do you want to give your impression first? And then I'll make up my answer. *(laughter)*

Connie: I felt a real command to raise one hand or the other, and I was keenly aware the whole time that I wasn't doing it, as far as I know. And I just had to allow that to be, but it was real uncomfortable, 'cause it seemed that that became the criterion of the trance; so I was going along with everything else on *one hand kind of dissociative* . . . *(laughter)*

Gilligan: I hope the relevance of that to *the issue at hand* is clear. Quite seriously, one of the things that you want to do—first of all, I introduced a lot of suggestions, not knowing exactly how the person is going to respond to them, and rightfully so, because people, I think, really are unique and will respond according to what's appropriate for them at the moment. This process that I am talking about, reversing certain patterns, is just one of a number of different ways of communicating that idea that I was seeding throughout the entire time, about establishing different patterns, that there's an expectancy of one thing happening, and a real intense hoping that one thing would happen. Yet I was talking about reversal of patterns. Now there were some ideomotoric responses in the hand, not a full hand levitation, and that really doesn't concern me. In fact, it's very nice response that can be utilized, because in the goal state that Connie has, there's going to be plenty of frustrations encountered. So a question becomes: How can I utilize their response as part of the therapeutic goals that are set up? And so, it's a good way to distract and orient and focus their attention, displace the failure onto the hand so that they can work independently at the same time. And also keep them aware, hoping something is going to happen if . . . and begin to teach them to have dissociated awareness, which was one of my prime goals here.

Bob Pearson: I think most of you know who I am. I followed Milton Erickson around like a little puppy dog for many years. And let me say to this group, that you have just witnessed the finest example of the embedded metaphor on a spontaneous basis that I have seen in many many years. Thank you, Steve.

Gilligan: Thanks, Bob.

(Applause)

Gilligan: Well, I think that's a good place to end. *(laughter)* Thank you all very much.

Commentary

Stephen G. Gilligan, Ph.D.

My initial contact with Connie as a volunteer subject came the day before the demonstration. She was among several individuals at the conference who asked if they could serve as the subject. She reported having attended a large 5-day training course of mine in New York City earlier in the year, and expressed an interest in using hypnosis to help her pass some upcoming comprehensive exams in psychology. I selected her because her goal seemed straightforward and addressable within a single session, and because she seemed to be a good hypnotic subject.

The Initial Interview

We met later that day for an initial interview. My thinking was organized around three basic questions: 1) What does she want? 2) What does she perceive as resources and obstacles to what she wants? 3) What are her customary patterns (of thinking, acting, feeling, etc.)?

What she wanted was clear and simple: to pass her comprehensive exams in psychology. She thought this would entail being able to prepare effectively, to relax during the test, to develop an experiential state (e.g., trance) optimal for test performance, to integrate diverse areas of learned information, to relieve any anxiety, and to still "inner chatter."

Among her resources were an excellent hypnotic ability, a solid knowledge base (that is, she knew the material), and a good history of taking tests. Her perceived limitations included a fear of failing, anxiety about integrating multiple areas of learned information, and a self-castigating internal dialogue. Other patterns included an attentional style of intense focused absorption, modest body catalepsy while thinking, and skills of dissociation.

Planning the Session

Once relevant information had been gathered, the next step was to think about how it could be used as the primary basis for the hypnotherapeutic work. Following this basic Ericksonian principle of utilization, I first translated each identified goal, resource, obstacle, and life pattern into a "simple idea" or "resource frame," then contemplatively identified various hypnotic phenomena and stories that would exemplify these ideas in a therapeutic fashion. This included jotting down the following:

1) *You have the ability to prepare at an appropriate rate* (stories: stretching and warming up for martial arts, students wanting to do too much too fast; hypnotic processes: interspersal of counting).
2) *You can relax during test* (stories: hypnotic absorption during writing of dissertation, "reducing chatter" by shifting from typewriter to computer; hypnotic processes: deep relaxation, hypnotic alteration of sensation).
3) *You can develop lucid dissociational awareness during test* (stories: Zeig's glider plane rides, lucid dreaming research; hypnotic processes: spatial dissociation, ideomotoric responses, hypnotic and, posthypnotically suggested, nocturnal dreams).
4) *You can integrate and reorganize many different areas of learning* (stories: computer "document link" processes, friend's medical exams, learning martial arts combinations; hypnotic processes: bodily dissociation of parts, with consequent reintegration into whole body experience).
5) *You can reduce anxiety and inner chatter* (stories: strategies of pain control; hypnotic processes: confusion and deep trance).

This list indicated a basic plan for the session: to hypnotically convey that each aspect of the target situation was an unconscious resource or ability that could be used and expressed in a variety of therapeutic ways. In other words, the hypnosis would revolve around affirming, activating, and making flexible each of the subject's relevant processes so that she could discover her own way of passing the exam. Of course, the plan was considered suggestive rather than mandatory; it was assumed that the actual hypnotic communications would include only some of these ideas, stories, and processes, while also including other references that arose "spontaneously" during the exchange. In this way, the plan was focused, yet not rigid, allowing coherence but also creativity.

Getting Started

By the time we began on the following afternoon, I felt well prepared. Setting my sheet of notes on a chair next to me, my first concern was to experientially connect with myself and with Connie. This is always my initial intention, since the effectiveness of my hypnotic work seems to depend in large part on the presence of an "interpersonal trance" (see Gilligan, 1987).

The presence of a large audience helped to focus my attention inward, and as my body became hypnotically absorbed, I extended my field of nonverbal awareness to include Connie. The sense of nonverbal connectedness with myself and with the client is essential in my work; without it, I would not feel sufficiently grounded to trust "unconscious" processes to "do their thing." When I am connected in this way, images and words seem to "come to me," rather than being effortfully created by my analytical processes. Whenever I feel stuck or otherwise off-center, I shift attention immediately to reconnecting with this nonverbal interpersonal field. I consider it much more important to therapeutic success than what is being said verbally.

It was not difficult to establish a sense of experiential absorption with Connie. As we nonverbally connected, I became intensely curious about how trance would develop, how her conscious processes could be paced and depotentiated, and how the central intention of passing the comprehensive exams could be hypnotically addressed in a variety of helpful ways.

Developing Trance

After asking a few preliminary questions to establish the purpose of our work together, I decided to develop trance via questions regarding previous trance experiences. Connie adjusted her posture and developed mild catalepsy, which I utilized by introducing the general idea of hypnotic dissociation and the specific suggestion of ideomotor finger response. She responded positively to this suggestion, which I ratified and framed as an instance of unconscious autonomy.

This process of unconscious responses was then extended to the areas of tunnel vision and body sensation. These suggestions were made because it seemed that she was already developing such responses; that is, her bodily catalepsy and fixed eye focus were outer indicators of inner bodily changes and visual alterations.

This initial interchange is typical in that the suggestions for hypnotic phenomena are primarily requests for the subject to amplify already occurring experiential responses. Thus, the hypnosis is elicited rather than imposed. This makes it easier for the therapist and more therapeutic for the client.

Introducing Ideas

A major purpose of developing trance in therapy is to enhance receptivity to new ways of thinking and behaving. Thus, Connie's development of trance indicated to me that she was ready to receive key ideas and suggestions. Much of the demonstration can be seen as involving the hypnotic communication of such ideas. Typically, an idea was emphasized (e.g., "You have the ability to integrate different areas of learning") and then an experiential example in the form of a story or a hypnotic phenomena was provided. These two levels of hypnotic suggestion serve to emphasize a general ability while also providing multiple experiential reference structure for expressing that ability.

One of the key ideas in hypnotherapy is that an idea becomes therapeutically potent only when it is experientially sensed as significant—when it is translated into some personally meaningful event. In this view, a major purpose of hypnosis is making ideas "come alive" in the body, so that they become realized in actual expression.

Utilizing Ongoing Responses

To ensure this "felt sense" of the presented ideas, the hypnotherapist needs to observe and utilize the subject's ongoing responses. One way to do this involves periodically "pacing" nonverbal responses ("You're doing this," "You're doing that"), thereby including the subject's body as an integral part of the conversational field.

A related technique is language suggestions in terms of already occurring responses. For example, at the beginning of the session Connie developed ideomotoric finger movements, so I emphasized how she could "wait [weight]" on the one hand and "recognize" things on the other hand. At another point, Connie moved her head, whereupon I noted how she could let her "unconscious do the learning . . . make the adjustment . . . head down, up, over to areas of learning that were going to be important."

A third technique is to observe bodily responses indicating analytical movement (e.g., arhythmic movements, eyebrow furrowing) and respond with techniques that depotentiate such interference with hypnotic processes. This was a major purpose in periodically using the overloading and confusing statements involving numbers and rapid shifts of topics. Such communications were designed to ensure that Connie didn't try to figure things out consciously, but rather would allow her unconscious mind to do the learning while in trance.

Concluding Remarks

While the above remarks suggest a great deal of thinking and strategizing on my part, it is important to emphasize that my actual experience during this hypnotic session (and most others) is decidedly unanalytical. While I train myself rigorously and try to prepare well for each client, the actual work is characterized by a deep sense of being an observer-participant. My interest is in discovering a cooperative partnership both with my unconscious and with the client so that the negotiated goals of the relationship can be realized in some unique and mutually satisfying fashion. Preparation and hard work is essential in this regard, but so is creativity and trusting the unconscious. When a balance between these two is realized, effective therapeutic work is often the result.

I believe that this happened with Connie. The videos clearly indicate the development of a therapeutic trance in both of us, and follow-up reports were equally satisfying. Specifically, Connie passed her exams with high marks and is now a practicing therapist.

Reference

Gilligan, S. G. (1987). *Therapeutic trances: The cooperation principle in Ericksonian hypnotherapy.* New York: Brunner/Mazel.

Commentary

Jeffrey K. Zeig, Ph.D.

The therapeutic use of indirect (multilevel) communication is probably *the* outstanding contribution Milton H. Erickson made to the health sciences. Therapeutic anecdotes were often a vehicle in which multilevel messages could be embedded. One striking example is Erickson's case of Joe and the tomato plants, where on the social level he discussed how a tomato plant grew, while on the psychological level he interspersed suggestions of pain control.

Embedded within a story (which could be something as commonplace as the growth of a seed into a tomato plant, or the process of a child learning to write the letters of the alphabet), Erickson used hypnotic language, including presuppositions, embedded commands, misspeaking, confusion technique, nonverbal methods, symbolic communication, directed truisms, and word-plays, to build a wealth of positive associations to elicit from within the patient's personal history—resources (previously unrecognized learnings) to accomplish therapeutic goals. When sufficient associations were elicited, salutary changes in behavior would be forthcoming because of ideodynamic effect whereby thoughts become actualized in behavior. For example, when one thinks about a lemon, one can begin to salivate. This ideodynamic effect is especially strong during trance.

If Milton Erickson was the inventor of therapeutic multilevel communication, Stephen G. Gilligan is the poet laureate. In this particular therapy, Gilligan is extraordinarily facile at guiding associations by weaving psychological-level messages within anecdotes and through using hypnotic language. Gilligan is confident, witty, and respectful of the patient with whom he works. His concentration is intense and approaches the remarkable concentration of Erickson. Careful study of this transcript will provide even the expert in Ericksonian techniques the opportunity to learn more about the language of hypnosis. More than that, the tape needs to be viewed to experience the wealth of nonverbal techniques that Gilligan uses to provide therapy. It is no wonder that Erickson's long-time student, Robert Pearson remarks at the end of the tape that this is the "finest example of embedded metaphor I have seen in many years."

There is an additional aspect of the technique of hypnotically embedding messages that has not received as much attention in the literature as it should. One of the "laws" of communication is that the effectiveness of therapeutic messages should be judged by the response of the subject, not merely by the cleverness inherent in the communication. Erickson used one-step-removed methods in concert with *eliciting responsiveness*. During the initial phase of induction, Erickson would build responsiveness to multilevel communication. For example, to elicit eye closure, Erickson might have suggested, "The next time I say 'now' . . . close your eyes . . . NOW!" Erickson often hesitated and softened his voice when he said the words, "Close your eyes," to make them a command. He would gradually "train" patients to respond to such subtle messages. Also, he would use cues that were more overt and perhaps confusing, as in the example above where the second "NOW" unexpectedly followed as both a pregnant command and as an intended indirect cue. Usually, Erickson would not proceed with therapeutic multilevel techniques until he demonstrated, during induction, observable responsiveness to general indirect suggestions. It was as if demonstrated responsiveness to general indirect techniques was a cue that the induction period of therapy was over and the therapeutic period of therapy was to begin.

Erickson often discriminated between the induction phase and the utilization phase of treatment, but he never clarified what signaled the end of induction and the beginning of utilization. Here is one way of making a distinction: When demonstrable response is garnered to the multilevel communication during induction, induction is over. It is as if the patient indicates: "Okay, I'm open to working with you. The door is open to my constructive unconscious. I will let you influence me." Therefore, Erickson would work during induction to elicit to the maximum extent possible the patient's responsiveness to minimal cues. Once initial responsiveness to indirect methods was established, the, therapy could begin.

In Gilligan's techniques, one can see the technique of building responsiveness to minimal cues. For example, early in the induction, Gilligan closes his eyes in a suggestive way. Subsequently, the patient blinks in response to Gilligan's cue and eventually closes her eyes. The importance of building responsiveness to minimal cues before eliciting therapeutic associations cannot be overemphasized. Casting seed onto the ground is not apt to lead to a good harvest unless the ground has been adequately tilled and fertilized.

Hindsight being 20-20, there are other options for treatment that could be pursued. For example, in this phase of his development, Gilligan emulates his mentor by using Erickson's voice tone and rhythm of speech. When Gilligan met Erickson, Erickson was an infirm man with a speech defect due in part to the residuals of polio. Gilligan modeled Erickson as a way of learning his teacher's methods. In retrospect, it might be more beneficial to use his own voice rather than Erickson's. As Gilligan has evolved over the years, he *has* developed his own voice.

Also, there is some overload for the patient. There is no possible way she can absorb, even unconsciously, all the multilevel messages Gilligan provides. A more targeted intervention may have been just as effective. Moreover, it would have been good to have some "follow-through." Gilligan's setup and intervention is masterful, but, perhaps due to the limitations of time, we do not get to see the follow through. For example, there could have been some "process instruction," perhaps through another story, at the end of the induction to provide suggestions for how to use the elicited resources. Alternately, there could have been some "future pacing" in which she practiced using some of the resources via mental rehearsal.

A final critique has to do with Gilligan's alembical method. If the masterful use of complex multilevel technique is necessary for successful treatment, we are in trouble, because only a few can aspire to Gilligan's poetic use of language and techniques of influence.

Motivating Action with Hypnotherapy for a Client with a History of Early Family Violence

Stephen R. Lankton, M.S.W.

My demonstration today is a rather open-ended one. It's Motivating Action with Hypnotherapy, which I thought was a broad-enough topic for us to be able to grasp it. I interviewed my potential client yesterday, and she will be my client today.

We talked a bit about the possibility of doing this and the usefulness of doing this, but not specifically about what we would really want to accomplish. I thought we would save that for the discussion now. I can't tell you ahead of time what is going to happen, so I guess we just better do it and find out. I'll tell you afterwards what happened if there are any questions.

Lankton: Would you be willing to tell us your age?

Linda: Sure; 42.

Lankton: When I discussed it with you, you had something in mind. It had a bit to do with self-effacing comments and your general motivation of yourself being inhibited by that. Could you say a little about it?

Linda: That I have a real strong desire to not be self-effacing. But somehow or other I have a lot of words and sentences that are strong that keep that kind of behavior coming professionally and personally.

Lankton: And even while you begin to talk on it, your reflection on it makes you sort of sad about this state of affairs or something. And you wish it wasn't that way. Am I reading into your sentences saying that you are unhappy about that?

Linda: I am unhappy about that. That's right. I'd like to change that.

Transcript of a demonstration given in Phoenix, December 1988.

Lankton: I would like to change it, if it were me. I'm not quite sure what your motivation is for changing it. Why do you want to? Woody Allen does fine with it.

Linda: I've thought of going into pictures. *(laughs)*

Lankton: You've thought of going into pictures? *(laughs)* So, keeping it might not be a bad idea if you could do that, but you don't have any contracts right at the moment. *(laughs)*

Linda: No. *(laughs)*

Lankton: And that's why we're doing this, then.

Linda: It is really unhelpful for me! *(laughs)*

Lankton: This is a tape screening. This is your screening for the movies. Is that . . .

Linda: *(laughs)*

Lankton: But what is your motivation for getting rid of this self-effacement? How do you imagine your life would be improved somehow if you did?

Linda: I wouldn't be, um, I would be able to be less afraid about being in groups and more able to receive credit when people try to give it to me. I would be able to teach easier without it being traumatic. I mean, those are the things I am doing.

Lankton: And your tears that you have here, you don't have those usually? It's just when somebody talks to you about it?

Linda: Or just when I talk about it. *(clears throat)*

Lankton: I guess you don't do it that much, then because then you would be crying.

Linda: No, not that much.

Lankton: I am going to present a paper that suggests that you ask questions like this to somebody, and in a way I am hesitant a little bit here to do it because when a person is self-critical and you start asking comments like "How or why in the world do you think you could change that," it is so easy for you to take the posture of "Well, maybe he is right' he's implying that I can't, and that's what I thought all along." So I don't know just how to ask you the question: Do you think you can change that?

Linda: Well, I've been working hard at it. I don't know.

Lankton: How are you doing? Are you succeeding?

Linda: Not very well. *(laughs)* No. I mean I was producing different behavior, but . . .

Lankton: But you have only two options. If you said anything other than "absolutely perfectly" you'd be . . . and if that is the case, then you wouldn't be here.

Linda: That's right.

Lankton: So evaluating your progress is something you better not do?

Linda: It's hard. That's right.

Lankton: Well, what do you suppose is the central element that . . . I imagine I am the way I am, you are the way you are, because of our . . . way that we remember the past, at least. We blame the past for the ways we are doing this stuff, or we credit the past for the ways we are doing it. What do you blame or credit for how come you are self-effacing?

In some ways I reckon it's a real strength that helped: kept you somehow from getting more punishment than you expect you might have gotten. And by keeping yourself self-critical, you've anticipated punishment and maybe removed some of the actual punishment that you would have gotten; so in a way it's been real handy, and it's sort of a survival strength. But why in the hell did you do it in the first place?

Linda: You mean as a child?

Lankton: I guess, yeah.

Linda: Well, I don't think I would have seen it as self-critical as a child. I grew up in a real difficult home. Um. I learned to watch.

Lankton: There may be some things you don't want to say about that, in fact. Is that true?

Linda: Well . . .

Lankton: There may be difficulties in the home, may be more than you want to talk about here.

Linda: Lots of violence, and the things that go with it. So . . .

Lankton: And why self-critical? How come that got in there? Why not like just a constant dialogue like "Jesus, I survived another day!" instead of self-critical? How do you suppose that part got in?

Linda: I don't know. I am one of seven siblings, and nobody's got that piece.

Lankton: Are you the oldest? So I suspect you took some responsibility for the others?

Linda: Yes, quite a lot.

Lankton: Ya. Well, I'm only asking that to get kind of a feel and to help other people get a feel, too, for um . . .

I would like to use the hypnosis, which is our demonstration. We might/could talk for two hours and really get something useful just by talking. I wonder what we could accomplish that would be useful in trance. That's what I would like to attempt to do. And I know that you will seek further help and so on afterwards, to the extent you need it, and you are capable of doing that.

So, with that sense of it in the background, I'd like to sort of arbitrarily move to the trance. It's not exactly the moment I'd do it in my office. I think I'd find out a few more things that you might want to tell me. Is there something that you *do* want to say?

Linda: No.

Lankton: Is there something that you'd like to not say?

Linda: *(laughs)* Yes.

Lankton: Why don't you start at the bottom of the list where it's the least threatening?

Linda: Ohhhh. *(laugh)* Nooo.

Lankton: Is there anything you think I should know that you don't want to say—that if I knew it, I would be more helpful, but you don't want to say.

Linda: That um . . .

Lankton: Well, you don't have to. I just mean is there something that . . .

Linda: No.

Lankton: So you kind of think that I am going to be able to be helpful even not knowing all that stuff.

Linda: I think so.

Lankton: Oh great. *(audience laughs)* Well, if I am helpful, it'll be helpful in the sense that it will be a springboard for you to do something for yourself, of course. And I know you have been ignoring the group somewhat; so why don't you ignore them a little more by closing your eyes. 's a good idea. Are your feet comfortable?

Linda: Yes.

Lankton: And our volume's okay?

Audience: No, speak louder.

Linda: Do you want my mike? My mike is probably better.

Lankton *(to audience):* Thanks for saying so.

Lankton: You go into a trance in your own way, fo course, and in your own time into the depth that is appropriate for you. And, although you may have your eyes open in the trance, you may begin by closing them. Sooner or later the sense of concentrating your attention and becoming comfortable, by letting your conscious mind focus "in" on certain thoughts that are least distressing for you, so that your unconscious can have some freedom to play with other thoughts, entertain other ideas, investigate experiences. You can lean back in the chair all right, or is that a problem?

Linda: *(leans back in chair)*

Lankton: One of the things that I sometimes ask people to do in a trance is to dissociate their experience in trance from everything else—to never have the generalization of the successful experience in the trance—not to anticipate having it, not to worry about having it. Just let this experience be all by itself, life standing on the observation deck of the Eifel Tower. Thinking about all that history, and you're not a part of it.

Like walking through the Louvres and thinking, "I'm glad I didn't have to paint all those emperors." You can stand in front of Michaelangelo's works, and it makes you proud to be a human being. And you know you couldn't do it, maybe no one ever again could do it. And it doesn't diminish it for one moment. And it doesn't diminish you for a moment.

And often the more relaxed a person becomes, the more they go into trance. I like to think about those situations where I was all alone, hiding under a cardtable, pretending I was the Lone Ranger, or running through the mud behind my house, pretending I had landed on the moon.

One person that I know had the fantasy of sending an android to school. He kept all controls in the attic, and when it was time to go to school, he slipped into the attic and sent the android out in his place. And from the safety of that distance, he had moments to think about what to say, consult books, and talk into the microphone, and the android would say the right words. *(long pause)*

I had many hours in a sensory deprivation tank once, when I lived in Jackson, Michigan. And for a year and a half or so, I'd slip into the man's house every night, an' he left it in his basement and gave me a key. And I learned to float in the water clock *(long pause)* and think of myself as totally disconnected from everything else. I could review the events of the day and turn on and turn off different sensorium, and my body was just there floating. It's like skin diving, scuba diving. There's a great deal of visual attention that has very little to do with what you're doing. And your body is just floating there. And for me trance is like all of those things. I've been very sleepy at the back of the movie theater. And I don't know why all the other people bothered to come. And so your conscious mind may think of various images like that in order to aid your unconscious mind. And my job is a person who can help by stimulating your conscious and unconscious thoughts in ways that could be of use to you.

Someone asked me about confusion and its role in therapy. I really doubt that you could fail to misunderstand confusion anymore than he does at those moments that he is certain of something. And I hope that you'll be very certain only of the fact that you are there in the chair and you are alone there and somehow you're not. Your cheek muscles are relaxed, there's a half-smile on your mouth, your rapid eye movement has decreased, you swallow reflex has slowed, you're breathing deeply from your stomach.

And to the extent that you begin to think about things that are relevant to you, there's no reason to move. I began by pointing out that I would like someone in trance to have the experience that what happened to them here is simply for now and for no other time. And I would like you to go into trance deep enough that, if it would be all right with you, to have an experience that you can have isolated from all other parts of your learning and thinking. Maybe you can think of a poem, and you will never remember it again. Or, you can have an experience that you don't particularly need to give yourself credit for or hold it against yourself ever again. This trance is a vacation from real life.

When I did a demonstration in Phoenix in 1983, there was a woman who had had back pain for 40-some years, and during the trance it was entirely gone. And I asked her to make sure that it would come back again after the trance was over so that, while she could remember that it had been gone, it didn't need to influence her real life in any way, unless she wanted it to.

There's another problem in telling metaphors to people in trance, and that is: Who will the person identify with? I think it would be perfectly legitimate for you to identify with everybody I talk about in the metaphor. I might talk about my daughter and my conduct with my daughter. I'd like you to identify with me. I'd like you to identify with my daughter. After all you can't really understand the situation that occurs to the people in the metaphor unless you have projected into it. It is reasonable to assume that you would project into both parts of it. I don't know if you have ever though about holding yourself as a little girl. Everyone sooner or later has the idea. Your conscious mind may have flirted with the idea and allowed your unconscious to have the experience a little bit. Maybe your conscious mind has had the experience a little bit and allowed your unconscious to flirt with the idea.

Sometimes Alicia will come into the office when I'm working, and I'm typing at the keyboard. She crawls up underneath my elbows and gets right in the middle of things. She says, "Hold me, Daddy." And what does a parent do? I say, "OK." and then I tell her what I was typing about and she listens and, after awhile, stroking her hair, she crawls away.

I remember on day at a workshop, she came and and she got up on my lap and she said she wanted to go, and I said, "We'll go in a minute. Go play." And then a couple of minutes had passed, and she came back and she said, "Daddy, you said we would go into a minute and it's been a minute." And I said, "All right, I have to go now. I have to keep my word." And I wonder how it makes a child feel, where you'd feel it on your face. What would happen with regard to your heart rate, your breathing rate, your feeling of your musculature, your sense of self? You learn it, it becomes a part of you. You bring it with you the next time you walk into the living room, 'n' crawl over on the couch, 'n' sneak up on my lap, 'n' crawl up on my neck, and say, "I just want to sit here for a while, Dad." And sometimes she says, "Daddy Honey," and then she *knows* that I am going to let her sit there. When she falls asleep in my arms, I put her in bed sometimes, trying so carefully not to wake her up.

One day the other week, she came out of the bedroom and said, "Mommy, you said you were going to lie down with me." Carol was so happy to be able to finally watch some television show, but she jumped up and said, "I will darling," and lay down with her. It only took a few moments before she had fallen asleep, and Carol did get to watch the show. And then sometimes I am up in the middle of the night. I always go past and make sure that she is covered and not cold.

There are a lot of ways that we can have feelings. Children learn to feel brave by pretending—pretending that they are Superman. And I remember the phrase "You can pretend anything and master it." All those children learn to play guitar; they pretend they are already a rock star; they pretend they are already able to play piano concertos. And not only is there no harm in pretending, it is very good rehearsal to make a space somewhere inside for that new feeling to develop. And how about dressing up like you're older when you're just a child? And pretending you can ride you bicycle "zoom" down the highway. And you are only riding a little cart around the living room floor.

Then you can think about my daughter and you can have those experiences. What is memory anyway except imagination? So go into trance to a depth necessary to allow you to have the imagination of the memory. Feeling that degree of safety and comfort, with the agreement that if you have it now, it's disconnected from everything. It's a trial period. It has no meaning. There's no threat that it will generalize into the rest of your life. Just like an ant digging a little bitty tunnel down into the sand and making a great big hole in which he can live, or a little rabbit that makes a little burrow, down a little thin hole up to the earth. But inside the burrow, who knows what that little rabbit is doing? Maybe just storing jars of honey before that Pooh Bear comes to visit.

And let the feeling of safety be something that you feel more now than you ever felt before. Know what it's like for your little finger to feel it, for your ankle. Feel the skin temperature changes with it. And know that your conscious mind needn't even remember it, but that you have made an agreement that you are going to the depth of trance necessary to have th experience now more than you have ever had it. And let it radiate to the tips of your fingers. Let it radiate out your fingers and toes. Ooze safety, security, belonging, in a way you most imagined that my daughter probably does. And then I want you to keep it constant for the next five minutes, with the agreement that if there is any difficulty for you having that experience, you can be fully assured that you won't have it again after the trance is over. It's just a little experiment.

You can say to your conscious mind or your unconscious mind, "Oops, it was just a mistake, like the Xray"—like the discovery of the transistor. But, rather than pull it out of the wastebasket, you can leave it in there. And now memorize and hold onto it. Does it feel good?

Linda: *(slight head nod and big smile)*

Lankton: I want you to do three things with it. I want you to open our eyes for a moment, and hold onto it. And close them and know that you were able to open you eyes and hold onto it. Is that correct?

Now, I want you to do the second thing and look at the group while you hold onto the feeling. All those shadowy figures out there from Jung's unconscious. Almost in the darkness. Makes it perfect to project onto them and see what you project onto them, while you feel that feeling. Can you say? What do you see?

Linda: That they . . . they look friendly.

Lankton: They look friendly? Accepting? They are happy that you are having feelings?

Linda: I think so.

Lankton: Now close your eyes again and memorize that, knowing that you can forget all about it after the trance if you like.

And now the third thing I would like you to do is to open your eyes and recover that precious feeling, knowledge, memory, awareness, projecting what you see onto the faces, knowing what that means, holding onto that feeling of safety, comfort. And now I want you to try really, really hard to have any self-effacing thoughts that you can have. Try to hallucinate on top of this scene that you see detrimental aspects and memories from your family-of-origin while holding onto this feeling and watching the group. Let your own hallucination intermingle. Try to have that memory, find out if you can really make it interfere or not with the experience you are having while you are looking at those people and using them as a way to remember your feelings. And don't listen to me for a moment, just go ahead and do that.

I want to mention to the group a rationale. This is reciprocal inhibition occurring. This is interesting kind of flooding in vivo. But it is not flooding the anxiety-producing experience of the fear, it is flooding the anxiety-producing experience of the security.

Now let me repeat my instructions and make sure you did it the way I envision it. That you are holding onto a feeling of safety and belonging, you are looking at the group and they are reminding you of the experience somewhat, too. And so you know you are here having that feeling. And then you are trying very hard to remember fearful, anxiety-producing, self-critical-generating experiences from the past and see that shadowy memory at the same time.

Sometimes I work with people and I mention that they will do an experience in the trance and they'll gain an idea that they just won't be able to shake when the trance is over. Something will seize their mind as a useful concept or an idea and it will stay with them.

What are you experiencing as you do that?

Linda: That, um, they are not dangerous and, um, I'm not wrong.

Lankton: Would you mind trying a little harder to remember even worse experiences that made you, compelled you somehow, to think that you were wrong. Keep your eyes focused on them while you keep this feeling and (pause). 'Cause there are going to be times when your memories of the past are used to solve problems in the present, and you want to be sure that you've looked through all your memories of the past and that none of them will inhibit you, that they all will be some kind of aid to you in the future. It would be really nice if all those memories that you are thinking about reminded you, at some level, that actually you were trying really hard to feel bad, and failed at it.

So I would like you to try so hard to feel bad while you are holding this feeling and looking at the group that you become aware that you failed at feeling bad. And maybe criticize yourself for that.

Linda: (laughs)

Lankton: Now, there's a mixture of happiness here and sadness a little bit. But the happiness is stronger, or not? Can you say what you are thinking of, what the memories are?

Linda: Of, um, with my sister and, um, of not being able to help the kids and, of, um, my brother dying, um, and things not getting better, and my not being able to help them, even as an adult, enough, um, of . . .

Lankton: What are you feeling while you are telling me this and looking out? Are you looking at the people?

Linda: Uh-huh. I am feeling, um, surprised . . .

Lankton: About?

Linda: I don't, I don't think they think I'm bad, or . . .

Lankton: Is that . . .

Linda: New!

Lankton: . . . different or something?

Linda: Uh-huh!

Lankton: You would have thought that if you . . .

Linda: Ya.

Lankton: then how do you feel besides surprised?

Linda: Comfortable.

Lankton: Is there anything else that you would like to feel comfortable about remembering? There's a lot of violence in the world, there's incest, there's self-mutilation, there's irrational violence that has no definition . . . and look at the people as you do, realize that you are here having this experience, and you are really trying to remember something that would make you feel bad. *(long pause)* Is there anything else? Is that all of them? There's always more. But if the ones you thought of are the worst of them, then the others are sort of inconsequential by comparison. Have you thought of the worst ones?

Linda: Uh-huh, out of the ones you talked about.

Lankton: So that's the third thing I wanted you to do. Now close your eyes again and *know* what you've done, just for now. You could look at it in a lot of different ways. You've really made contact with people, and in doing that held onto an experience that was pleasant. And it has a lot of different meanings in different ways.

One time in karate class, I accidently turned around doing a kata and broke some tile with my hand, months before I expected to be able to break tiles with my hand. And I remember riding down the driveway on my bicycle, certain that my parents or my sister was holding the back of the bicycle. Training wheels had been removed. And when I got to the bottom of the drive, I had made it the whole way, and I turned around to say I made it. And there wasn't anybody there. I went the whole way by myself. I don't know how it happened, but I accidently learned to swim one day. I left poor old Joe Kuchar in the shallow end of the pool and joined the others in the deep end. There are so many things that we do by accident that we didn't plan on ever having connect to the rest of our life.

I don't usually tell fantasy stories, but there is this one story that I was thinking about that has to do with this young man named Sheath, who lived in the desert before the age of technology, before animals were known through classification, when the world was quit a mystery. And he had lived kind of in isolation with a wall around him for a long time, in a city with a wall around it. It seemed perfectly reasonable. It was all he knew.

He had very few possessions, and he carried them with him most of the time: a key—didn't open any lock, a feather that he pretended was an eagle feather (which actually just came from a seagull that had gotten lost in the desert), a whistle that he hardly every used because when he blew it it didn't make any sound, and a crystal. He really liked the crystal. He wore it around his neck, but he was afraid he would lose it, so he dept it in his pouch.

And they weren't worth much to anyone, but they were all the possessions he had—except a towel. "It's a rough world and you have to know where your towel is." Ford Prefect said that in Douglas Adam's *Hitchhikers Guide to the Galaxy*. One of the best tips, I think, and this was applying to Sheath.

He left the town in his youthful exuberance, filled with delusions, one day and wandered out into the desert to see what he could find. And he didn't find anything—except more desert. And after he had been gone several days, (he wasn't quite sure of the number), he had his fill of sand and nothingness and he turned around and went back. But when he got back to where he came from, the city was gone.

His home was gone, and the fountain that he used to sit on was gone, and the wall he used to walk on was gone, and the people he talked to. And all of his childhood memories had been attached to these things. And they were all gone. His first thought was that he had surely gone to the wrong place in the desert. But upon further searching and watching the stars, he was sure he was in the right place. Whenever he did come upon another person and asked them, they didn't know anything of the city. So, he figured it was a conspiracy in which either all people who knew of the city had vanished with the city, or he simply hadn't come upon anybody yet who knew of the city.

His only alternative, it seemed, was to journey several days towards the North Star where the Magistrate who ran the large city was said to be a Magi, a wiseman of many talents, and maybe he could help him recover his way to his home. And when he finally arrived, the Magistrate gave him audience, heard his story, and said, "Yes, what we have here is a problem of the heart. And this will be a test of your heart." Sheath said, "You have had this kind of thing happen before?" The Magistrate said, "Well, it's always different in each case. And this one, of course, is unique. But one thing that is certain to me is that sometimes it's a matter of courage and sometimes it's a matter of wit, and sometimes it's humor, and sometimes it's love, and other times it's strength, or endurance. And for you it's a matter of the heart. And the tests that you have will be a test of your heart."

And Sheath said that he had no idea of how to pass any test of the heart. What could he possibly do? The Magistrate gave him the advice that he had learned to give many times before in similar situations. Sheath was to go back to the place from which he came, to go into this meditative state, and to "stay put in that situation until four things come to your mind four times. Whatever these objects are, gather them, bring them back here and your tests will be tests that will evaluate your ability to survive and prove or fail the test of the heart." And with that his granted audience was over. Sheath was to leave.

Sheath went back to where he had come from. He sat down and he meditated. But he didn't know many things, and he didn't own many, and he didn't have many. And, unfortunately, the only four things that came to his mind repeatedly were the key, the feather, the whistle, and the crystal. After a day and a half of trying to find his *true essence* he decided that was surely all that was going to come to his mind, and he set out with these four objects back to the Magistrate.

After an afternoon of walking in the desert, he was relieved to see a circus caravan come by and ask him if he would like to ride, and he said, "Yes, it would be wonderful to take a ride." Unfortunately, he had to ride in an empty cage. It was the only place there was any seating left. And he rode in the empty cage, jiggling and joggling along in the desert on wooden wheels. He fell asleep.

When he awoke all was still. And he thought at first, perhaps, that since it was dusk, maybe people were napping, and he was very quiet gathering his things. And then he discovered the door was locked in the cage, and he said, "Hey, guys, there has been a little mistake here." And there wasn't a sound, there weren't even the sounds of the animals, or the tambourines jingling. And he hollered louder, and he peeked, as best as he could. And he came to the conclusion that his cage had come separate from the caravan and he was alone, locked in the cage.

Then he knew it must be malice. These people were surely part of the conspiracy to hide the city. Then he thought maybe he had been robbed, but, no, he had his material with him. Maybe it was an accident. Maybe they didn't even know. Maybe he was left to his own devices. And somehow in all this thinking, he had grabbed a hold of the key. And as people will do, he had fidgeted the key into the lock. And to his surprise he opened the lock on the cage. He jumped out in such a hurry, he didn't realize that he lodged the key hopelessly in the lock! It wouldn't have come out if he'd thought to pull it out. So he continued walking across the desert, wondering how upset they would be to find that they had lost this cage, and perhaps remember that he had been in it, too.

Darkness and the night, which is usually absent of animals as far as he was concerned, suddenly became filled with animals. And in the darkness of the desert, the sound of growling and the footsteps seemed to be ominously close. He tried to whistle a little tune to pretend he wasn't afraid. But that didn't work. That just drew more animals closer. So he tried to be perfectly quiet, but he couldn't—his breathing gave him away. Finally, he was so frightened by the animals, he decided that what he better do is to call for help. Trying to call for help he found, as some children will do, that a scream just won't come out when your mouth opens up.

And he reached down and grabbed the whistle that never made any sound at all, and he blew it as hard as he could. And it made a loud shrill, almost outside of human range! And then everything was quiet except one thing—the sound of the pieces of the whistle hitting the ground. He blew it apart calling for help so loud. But there weren't any animals around. The shrill sound had blasted their sensitive ears. And he walked until morning.

He napped, and he walked further the next day. Finally he reached the gates of the city. Several miles from the Magistrate's office—there was a large city indeed—lying there in front of the gates of the city was a large beast. Fortunately, we don't know whether it was a dragon or a cyclops or just what it was because animals hadn't been codified back in those days. But it was much larger than the kind you would want to wrestle with in a dark alley.

And he was sure that it was an evil beast, and perhaps he would be devoured if he didn't sneak away. But then he wouldn't be able to complete his mission, find his city, recover his homeland, pass the test of the heart—whatever it was going to be. It was the creature that he know was evil and bad, and nasty and mean—carnivorous, no doubt.

Then he thought, "Maybe it's not. Maybe he is just a large hunk of sleeping flesh." And he reached into his pack to see if he had anything that could aid him. He had no tools, no magic, no weapons—he had a feather. And he reached over and tickled it with his feather. And the slumbering beast rolled a little bit. And he knew then if he kept tickling and kept nudging with that feather the beast might eventually—and sure enough it did—roll over, away from the entrance to the city. And so doing it trapped the feather in one of its armpits and pulled the feather from his hand.

Sheath went into the city now, about to have the victorious moment of seeing the Magistrate, and he reached in his pack and it dawned on him that he only had his crystal left. He had lost the key and his whistle and his feather. He looked at that crystal and he saw his reflection as he walked across the desert, he thought (the desert floor of the city), he thought how he had been walking for days to pass these tests of the heart, and now he was going to be a failure. He turned the crystal around and saw the different pictures of his face in despair—twelve facets of despair on his face.

Finally, he met the Magistrate. He told him of his failure, and the Magistrate congratulated him on the job well done. He had passed the test! Now, "How could this be," said Sheath? "I saw my face full of despair in the crystal." And the Magistrate, "Yes, you could have turned away, you could have denied, but you have a heart filled with *truth* and you saw it. And you could have thought that the beast was evil and malicious, but you thought it was humorous, and your heart passed the test of being a *light* heart. And you saw that the cage had come undone, and you could have thought that it was evil and malicious, but your decided that it was an accident, and you have the *capacious and forgiving* heart. And when the animals threatened you, you could have tried to be brave and pretend, but you have the *trusting* heart and you asked for help. And every step of the way you passed your test. Go back to where you came from now, and you will find, I think, free of delusion, that the home you look for is there. And to make a long story short, that's just what he did.

So when you come out of trance in just a moment, I would like to suggest that you keep an amnesia for whatever we have done here if you would like and know that you never have any responsibility to use the experience that you had here today. It was a vacation. You don't need to generalize it into the rest of your life, and change in anyway anything that you've done.

And know, too, that the woman that I worked with in 1983 let her back pain come back for a few days, and over the course of the next six months it went away entirely and is still gone five years later. Because you can use those kind of unconscious accidental experiences that occur to you, in your own way, at your own speed, and let your unconscious discover just how or *if* you'll use what you've done here today. Hi.

Linda: Hi.

Lankton: Do you want to realize that the group is back also? How do you feel?

Linda: Okay *(wiping her right eye with her left hand)*

Lankton: Is that a tentative one?

Linda: Ah, no. *(laughs)* I feel fine.

Lankton: You are looking like perhaps there's some, ah, is there more emotion now, is there some sadness again, I see.

Linda: No.

Lankton: Your voice is gone.

Linda: I know.

Lankton: Why?

Linda: I don't know. I was, I wasn't ready to finish.

Lankton: And you were ready to finish. You know, usually in a trance I mention you can go back to the experience that is unfinished and think about it when you are alone, or when you are in another trance, or when you dream at night, and complete any uncompleted ideas that you began in the trance. And I really should have said that. So I hope you will think to do that . . .

Linda: Yeah.

Lankton: . . . one way or another. Is there anything you want to say?

Linda: No thanks. It feels fine. (she looks off to the group, defocuses her eyes, and looks down to her right slightly)

Lankton: Well, thank you for participating. I think it might have been a helpful lesson in some ways to some of us, at least. Thank you, I believe we are done now.

Commentary

Stephen R. Lankton, M.S.W.

The client in this tape, Linda, had a history of physical and sexual abuse in her home. She is 42 years of age, lives alone, and had not married at the time of this therapy. She reported avoiding others due to self-imposed criticisms and thoughts that she was not acceptable. I had interviewed this client at length the previous day, and she had taken, at my request, an Interpersonal Checklist (Leary, 1957) self-report, which showed unusually high scores in the area depicting self-effacement. She specifically requested that the therapy be conducted to help her be more able to accept compliments.

The procedure used in this session is a tool that should be used cautiously in the therapy of incest victims and victims of family violence. It is designed to help reduce reliance upon denial as a defense. Therefore, clients need to be sufficiently interviewed and understood; it must be ascertained that potentials for suicide or other types of destructive behaviors do not exist. Furthermore, additional therapy should be arranged to follow the client after an intervention such as this. These considerations were taken and are mentioned in the session.

During the interview, the client revealed that she spent many years of her childhood trying, and as she saw it, failing to protect her younger siblings from the violence she suffered at the hands of her father. She indicated that she recalled historical events of what she believed to be her failures. She was unable to talk about herself without crying, and she commonly believed that others were unaccepting of her.

During the trance session, Linda demonstrated that she had the ability to project positive experiences onto others even while she remembered the most difficult of her memories of family violence. Four months after the therapy, she reported being surprised to find that she sought out and engaged in more social contact, including allowing others to touch her for the first time. What is more, the increased social contact occurred simultaneously with a great deal of criticism from a co-worker who was in disagreement or in competition with her. She stated that she was more aware of the incidents from her past and that she was not self-critical as a result of this increased awareness. She reported that she "opened up." As a consequence, she used subsequent therapy to do additional "difficult and painful" work involving aspects of her past that she refused to face or share with others before this session.

What I found most interesting about the session were three areas: 1) the method of dealing with social avoidance and post-traumatic stress; 2) the paradoxical restraint to prevent her from "failing" with any learning from the trance; and 3) the emphasis, with metaphor, on reevaluating her life as that of a person with a "good heart."

In the trance I helped her retrieve feelings of security and worth and then had her use them in small steps, in each of which she verified her success before proceeding. She kept the feeling of self-esteem with her eyes open while looking at others (who were looking at her), and she saw the others as accepting her. Finally, she continued to see others as accepting her while she "tried as hard as she could" to remember, in a sort of visual and auditory hallucination, a range of violent events from her past—the type, I assume, that typically intruded into her normal waking state and resulted in her self-criticisms and parataxic distortions.

I asked her, paradoxically, to make this session a respite from her normal life and not to feel that she had to learn from it in any way. She was just to let this be what it was, an interesting experience, separate from her life. I assumed that she would grasp at all experiences, including this one, that would help her growth. In this case, her consciously stated goal was accepting compliments. Unconsciously, of course, this may have had a myriad of meanings for her, but all must involve a higher evaluation of her self, a sense of safety and worth around others, and a movement toward others. In short, the things accomplished in this session must be part of the ability she sought to develop.

The reason for asking her to refrain from generalizing from the trance or trying to use the comforts and perceptual skills practiced in it was to reduce her anxiety. I did not want her to leave the session with an expectation from me or even from herself (stimulated by me) that she should use the experience in any discernable manner. Her evaluation of herself almost always reveals to her a less than acceptable performance and creates anxiety, subsequent depression, and withdrawal. There is a risk that this would happen no matter how carefully I worded a request for gradual improvement. In fact, if she were to leave with such an expectation, and conclude that she had not used it well "enough," the therapy would have resulted in yet another let down and source of anxiety.

She would be less likely to have anxiety about using the experience "well enough" if she were asked, repeatedly and with good reason, not to use it at all. While that sounds like a paradoxical directive, the goal is not to have her use it by telling her to not use it. Rather, the goal is to allow her the freedom not to use the therapy experience and, therefore, help allay her anxiety.

If she were to use the experience to help herself feel more comfortable getting compliments, being close to others, and motivating more work in therapy, etc., it would be preferable. But, if she were not to heed my directive and to, therefore, use the experience, it would be more likely due to her creative involvement with it than due to a performance demand or expectation from me. In conclusion, if she felt she had not gained from the trance experience, she would be free from additional anxiety—she was asked not to gain. So, this directive, developed over the course of the trance, sets up a relatively safe win-win position for her regarding freedom from anxiety that might otherwise have been stimulated by the therapy.

Finally, I told her a fanciful story concerning a person who felt he had little of value and who felt cut off from others. In the course of the story, the protagonist is pitted with a series of tests and the entire meaning and importance of his life is at stake. He seems to have failed at several tasks in the story until, in the end, it is seen that the behavior he considered failure at each step is really proof that he has passed a test of the heart. In fact, he is far better than he imagined in each case due to his limited, negative interpretation of his actions. In this story the protagonist is asked to see his life from a broader perspective—one in which he is a worthy and admirable person for his deeds.

I have reviewed this tape several times, and I really don't know what I would have done differently if I were to have a chance. But I conducted the session as hypnosis and therein, perhaps, lies a clue to what I might have done differently. That is, in a session in my office, not designed to simultaneously demonstrate hypnosis, I might not have used hypnosis. This client may have been able to profit from gestalt awareness and contact exercises. I believe I would have been inclined to use these viable options if I had not been destined to conduct this session as hypnosis. Yet, I am satisfied with the session and the client's reaction to it during and several months afterward.

References

Leary, T. (1957). *Interpersonal diagnosis of personality.* New York: Norton.

Commentary

Joseph Barber, Ph.D.

I am very impressed by the follow-up information we are given in this case. It is unusual in demonstration circumstances such as these to have follow-up data available, and it is pleasing that Lankton has provided this information. This tells us that the demonstration was more than an interesting and entertaining interchange. It tells us that something, for some reason not yet identified, created a significant and healthy and enduring change in the client.

I also have a response to the way Lankton responded to the stated goal of the client—to be able to better accept compliments. While such a goal certainly represents an understandable wish, Lankton's evaluation of the goal reflects his understanding that there may be underlying problems that need the client's attention. Lankton's initial evaluation included analysis of the Interpersonal Checklist, which revealed a significant deficit in self-esteem. His work with the client was clearly oriented toward ego-enhancing suggestions. These suggestions were certainly supportive, benevolent, and multifaceted.

When thinking about what I might do differently, I wonder if the complexity of the suggestions (or of their indirect character) is necessary. I wonder what the result would have been if Lankton had offered her suggestions of similar content, but in a simpler, more contactful way. Was it necessary for Lankton to go to such lengths? Might the client have been receptive to simpler contact? We cannot know, of course, what causes change in a client. It might be that these suggestions, created in just the way Lankton did, are responsible for the client's reported improvement in social contact. Or, it might have been something else. In any case, I probably would have been inclined to be more direct and less oriented to telling stories, much less so than I once was.

Aside from my differences with the theoretical basis for the successful work demonstrated here (which can otherwise be understood in the context of contemporary cognitive therapy), Lankton's work represents a profound empathy with the client's phenomenology and highlights the value of ego enhancement suggestions and benevolent attention, whether presented directly and simply or offered in the form of stories.

Solution-Oriented Hypnosis

William Hudson O'Hanlon, M.S.

Stan: I've got a sort of anxiety that I've had for the past couple of weeks.

O'Hanlon: Great. I'll take it.

(Stan: seats himself on the platform)

O'Hanlon: So you are supposed to be nervous being up here. Are you doing that?

Stan: A little bit. I'm okay so far.

O'Hanlon: A little bit. Okay. So tell me your first name.

Stan: Stan.

O'Hanlon: Okay, Stan, because they are doing videotaping, I assume that The Erickson Foundation has a release form. Usually when I do videotapes, there is a sort of permission form. They are doing video-taping and audiotaping, and so we'll have you sign a release if that's okay with you. If it isn't, we should find somebody else. You know this is sort of the fee you pay for being up here.

So, tell me a little bit. I guess I would like you to answer a few questions for me. Have you ever been in trance before, that you know about? Like this formal type? A few times? A lot of times?

Stan: I'd say once or twice.

O'Hanlon: Once or twice, okay. And the other thing is: If you could teach—it's a funny way to say it—if you could teach me how I could get anxious, how do you think you'd do it? I mean, I'd like you to teach me to be anxious. I'm a little hyperactive here, but I'm pretty comfortable. So . . .

Stan: Well, I haven't had much experience with it other than the past few weeks.

O'Hanlon: So this is sort of a new development.

Stan: I notice that your heart beats a little faster; it's like a hollow feeling.

Transcript of a demonstration given in San Francisco, December 1988.

O'Hanlon: A hollow feeling right there. Maybe if I could get my heart to beat a little faster, that would be good.

Stan: A little faster.

O'Hanlon: What else?

Stan: My voice is just a little bit, you know, tremulous.

O'Hanlon: A little quaver here and there—a tremulo here and there.

Stan: Let's see. You wouldn't want to sleep as much as you normally do. You'd wake up earlier.

O'Hanlon: You'd wake up earlier, and maybe I'd wake up and not go back to sleep in the middle of the night? Or just wake up early?

Stan: Sometimes waking up earlier—like an hour before you normally get up, and then starting to think about a problem that you have, almost in an obsessional way.

O'Hanlon: Going over it, and over it, and over and over it. Okay, that's pretty good. Yeah, and what would I be thinking about? Sort of, what I could do about it, or what I should have done about it, or maybe, am I going to be able to do this kind of stuff, or all of the above?

Stan: All of the above.

O'Hanlon: That would be good. And what else? Anything else in terms of . . .

Stan: Just worry, worry. You know, just like worrying a lot over some episode, or something you are going to say to somebody.

O'Hanlon: Anything in particular you know about that went by in the last few weeks, a particular project, or a particular situation that has gotten you sort of to focus more in that sort of way?

Stan: Uh-huh.

O'Hanlon: And anything you know you need to do that you haven't been doing?

Stan: Yeah, I need to talk more.

O'Hanlon: To talk more with a particular person? Or with other people about that situation? Or both?

Stan: I think to the person.

O'Hanlon: To the person. You need to get some feedback from the person?

Stan: Okay, good.

O'Hanlon: Great, and in the meantime, it would be a bit easier, and a bit nicer for you if you could come to it in a little more relaxed way, and still have the motivation and interest to go and talk to that person and clear up or try to clear up whatever you could clear up. In the meantime, it would be nice to sleep a little more, and be a little more comfortable. Okay, that's good.

Stan: Yeah.

O'Hanlon: All right, good. So when you've gone into trance before, how have you typically done it? Sitting in a chair?

Stan: Well, one time I was sitting in a chair.

O'Hanlon: Okay. Did you have your eyes open or your eyes closed?

Stan: *(questioning look)*

O'Hanlon: Do you wear contact lenses?

Stan: Yes. But that's not a problem.

O'Hanlon: Okay, you can close them.

Stan: Good.

O'Hanlon: All right, so I guess all other things being equal, let's just go into trance.

Stan: Okay.

O'Hanlon: That's right. At first I'll say that you can just allow yourself to be exactly where you are. There's no right way or wrong way for you to *go into trance*. Nothing particular that you need to do consciously to go into trance. Now you've been in trance before and I really don't know how *deeply* you've gone *into trance* before. But don't *go* any *deeper* than you need to go in order to make arrangements with yourself to *feel more comfortable, feel better*. And how will you know when you're that *deeply* in trance? Your conscious mind may have one thought about it, and your unconscious mind may be thinking something totally different. So just let yourself be exactly where you are. Initially, you could be consciously distracted by the sound around; you could be listening to the sound of my voice. But you don't really have to concentrate on anything. You can attend to whatever you're attending to. You can even be analyzing what I am doing, what I am saying. At the same time, you can be going into the kind of trance that is appropriate for you . . . in order to *feel more comfortable*, making whatever adjustments you need to for your *comfort*, your psychological *comfort*, physical *comfort*, emotional *comfort*, and finding a way to validate and support yourself for whatever experience you have right now. And open up the possibility that you are going to have, in a strange way, a sense of *more comfort* about the *discomfort* that you have. Just like you were relatively *comfortable* coming up on stage, even though you were a bit uncomfortable. It would be a sort of a nap of comfort that can include and support your experiences, your discomfort, and to be able to open up the possibility somewhere inside. You know exactly what to do to *be more comfortable*.

And one thing you already know how to do very deliberately, is to go and talk to a person that you need to talk to. You know that you need to say something, and maybe ask something. And while keeping yourself focused on that goal, or what's important for you to do, your body can support you enough by eliminating all the unnecessary anxiety.

While I was working with a woman who was on a certain medication that is very helpful for depression, the side effect was that it raised her blood pressure. The doctors wanted to take her off that medication as an antidepressant medication. But she was afraid that she would get so depressed without the medication that she'd become suicidal. So she really wanted to be able to have the very specific result of having her heart pump in a different way so her blood pressure readings would *go down—down to the level that was appropriate* for her. And after we did some hypnosis, she told me something that made me understand a lot better what her task was. She said, "You were talking to my *body* about blood pressure changes, about blood flow changes, but I think what my *body* really needs to *hear* is that my heart can *rest longer,* that my heart can *relax.*" And so I told her that she knew how to do that already. Because sometimes the blood pressure *had been down.* It was the lower reading that needed to come *down*—below 100 down to 90, and even below 90. So as I counted *down* from 100 to 90, I suggested that the *heart* could *rest* and *find the relaxation* that it needed, partly because the *rest* of her muscles had already learned how to *relax.* And the *heart* could be in a state of *dynamic relaxation,* for it would *relax just long enough* to do what was appropriate for that person—which might not be appropriate for anybody else.

And I remember going through some relationship difficulties myself, where I was hurt, something that happened in a relationship. And for a little while after that, maybe for a long while actually, I felt as if I put up sort of a shield or a barrier around my heart. It was obviously just a metaphor, but it had very real consequences for me. And then over the time after that, as I found environments that were safe and nurturing for me, I felt as if an outer crust was coming off *piece* by *piece* from around my heart, and that I found situations that I could trust. And at first it didn't happen *automatically,* but after a while it started happening *on its own.* Sort of *piece* after *piece* of that outer crust would come off, and there was a healed heart underneath. And to realize that I had more to do with that than the situation that I was in, and that when I put around that barrier, I was putting a barrier for myself to my access to my love, to my caring, to my openness.

So we can have metaphors for what happens inside of ourselves, sort of symbols and images. And you might be able to *find some image inside, some symbol inside* that symbolizes a time when you were *more comfortable,* or healing, or whatever other kind of idea that you have. Or maybe a symbol of your heart as a pump and just *slowing down* that heart rate, or filling up that hollow. Now if you can go into trance, you can *go to sleep.* I think that what I do sometimes is what I call a minitrance. A minitrance is just to get me back to by body's natural abilities to *respond biologically* to whatever the biological need is at the moment.

I do a lot of workshops. Occasionally, on the breaks in the workshops, I am in the bathroom at the same time the workshop attendees are; and I'm standing at the urinal and there's a lot of pressure. I'm the workshop's leader and I'm supposed to be cool, but maybe I get shy bladder every once in a while, so I found a technique that they don't know about that I do. I stare at the top of the urinal and I read the little logo or see the little silver part on top, and I go into a minitrance. It's like I just *get out of the way* and *let my body relax*, and *do what it needs to do*.

So if you just *let yourself go to sleep*. It's a bit like trance because at first when you start trance, you think, "Am I doing it right? Oh no, it's not going to work for me." You have all this sort of conscious mind chatter. At least most people do. And sometimes, *as you're continuing in trance*, you have some of that chatter. And at the same time, *experientially* you're becoming *involved* in being entranced. But there's a different *level*. And so it's a matter of just *allowing that experience* rather than making it happen. It's a matter of *letting yourself be* where you are. And making room for that experience of *going to sleep*. And also giving yourself permission to stay up if you stay up, and sort of *support yourself* while you are going through that *process*, rather than trying to manipulate yourself to *change* yourself. Get with the process.

There's a phrase that I've heard: "It's easier to ride the horse in the direction it's going." I heard another phrase, too: "Some people try to drive their cars by looking in the rearview mirror." It makes for a lot more crashes. So it's good to be oriented, I think towards where you are going, rather than where you've been. I saw a demonstration videotaped at one of the last big conferences where I attended a workshop. And the man was doing some negotiations with a couple, and at one point, the husband got way off the track and started complaining about something in the past. He said, "I want you to know." He said to the therapist, "I want you to know where I'm coming from." And the therapist said, "Actually, I'm not very interested in where you're coming from; I'm interested in where you're going to." So where would you like to go?

So to *orient your attention* to where you want to be, where you want to go, and then *allow* yourself to *move toward that*. Have your attention focused on where you want to be, where you are going, and then *pay attention* to where you are now. And make the connection between those two points. Maybe sometime in the *past* you can remember a *time* when you were *pretty comfortable*, maybe having taken a long hot bath—that kind of *comfort*, that physical relaxation *comfort*—or maybe being in a really nice space in your life, nice time, *feeling very content*, or not just content—happy, *good*. And the *muscles* seem to *respond to that*; the *breathing* seems to *respond to that*; the *heart* seems to *respond to that*.

And your *body* knows exactly what those *good feelings*, the feelings of *comfort* and *relaxation,* are like.

And you can make whatever *adjustments* you need to make in order to *feel comfortable now* and *in the future.* And how *deeply* you need to *go into that experience.* Now that *you've done that,* and how *quickly* will you know that *you've done that*? It won't be the first thing that you've *noticed* about the *changes.* And how will you know that it's going to *last*? That something has *changed* for you?

So when I go into trance sometimes, I *go into trance* and *come back* out a little; go into trance; it's like an ebb and a flow. Sometimes I *go all the way down,* but I just *follow my process* and *allow what happens to happen,* and I recommend that you *do the same.* Once I started doing a lot of trance, I *noticed* what would happen after a while. As I went into a *trance,* as I was doing *trance,* and then after a while as I *talked,* that little chatter in my mind would disappear—what I call my Howard Cosell voice in the back of my head. That Howard Cosell voice was always commenting on my experience or analyzing, or rehearsing things like you talked about. And one of the ways I noticed that I did was I just *focused* on what was *happening right now.* And I focused my attention on what I was *interested in.*

And usually when I am doing hypnosis for somebody else, I just focus on what they are *doing physically.* The responses that they are giving. And I notice that my concern with myself is diminished. That is, I am so much in *touch* with myself in some way that I don't *focus* on myself, my concerns, my needs so much. And I focus on someone else. My boundary seems to be *going out* in a *nice* way so that I've sort of included them in my space. Then, of course, there's a time when I *pull back into myself.* So you need to know when to expand the boundaries and when to pull them back. Sometimes I can understand your concern about talking to somebody else; it can be a risk.

I remember a story that Albert Ellis told some years ago about how, when he was in college, he was a shy kid. He was afraid of rejection, and at the same time—if you know Albert Ellis—a pretty horny little guy. He wanted to have some contact with women. And he wasn't the best looking guy on campus. He was a philosophy major, and he decided he needed to learn how to handle rejection philosophically. So he set himself a task of each month asking at least a hundred women for a date. Now, he lived in New York City so this was possible. And he got all the worst kind of rejections you could possibly imagine. "No way, I wouldn't go out with you if you were the last man on earth." "I'm sorry, I'm washing my hair on Friday night; oh yeah, I'm going to do it again on Saturday night—wash my hair." All sorts of rejections. And he had to learn to handle them without taking it personally. And also, he got a lot of acceptance. Some people just didn't know how to say no so they went out on dates with him. Some people decided that he was kind of cute—with his horn-rimmed glasses and his particular presentation. Some people were terrified of being without a date on Friday or Saturday night because of what it might say about them, so they went out on dates with him. And he ended up having dates almost every weekend.

And I sometimes tell people when they come into my office having just ended a relationship and maybe feeling bad about that, "Imagine that you went to the park every day and you fed the pigeons, and then one day you went to the park and you threw out the pigeon feed and the pigeons flew away." Now what some people do with that is they say, "Oh, I'm a shitty pigeon-feeder. I'll never find any pigeons to feed again. The pigeons must not like me. No pigeons will ever like me again." And these people get pretty depressed, pretty upset, scared. Sometimes they withdraw, isolate themselves, and don't communicate with people. And then there's another variety of people who say, "Those stupid pigeons don't know a good pigeon-feeder when they see one!"

But I'd say that you don't need to make conclusions about yourself or other people. Sometimes the pigeons just fly away. And it may have something to do with them; it may have something to do with the circumstance. But you don't really know for sure. So you can find some ways inside to make arrangements with yourself now and in the future to be as comfortable as you need to be, while continuing to take care of what you need to take care of, communicate what you need to communicate. And I've often found the anticipation of the thing is much worse than the thing.

I used to be a professional procrastinator. I'm still pretty good at it, but I've dropped down to amateur status. And I often find that thinking about doing the thing and worrying about it or avoiding it takes a lot more energy than sitting down and doing it. And the doing of it is rarely anywhere near what I was thinking it would be. Well, occasionally it is, but most of the time I was spending so much energy avoiding it, or worrying about it, or beating myself up about doing it. So, instead I always think of doing it, and starting it, and doing one little piece at a time, taking one little step, or sort of painting myself into a corner by promising that I'll have the paper done by a certain time. Yesterday I had a paper due early in the morning. At 8:00 I was up getting it printed out at the business center at the hotel. If I hadn't had that deadline, it could be another six months or a year before I'd get it done. So I think it's important to somehow figure out a way that you can take a step toward what you need to do, and get yourself into the process of doing it. Find the words that you need to say it in a way that's right for you.

And now, I just want to give you a minute or two of clock time—as much time inside as you need—to *do whatever you think you need to do to say whatever you need to say* to yourself, or just be with yourself, and let yourself float, drift, whatever . . . give yourself a minute or two, if you haven't already . . . I'm going to invite you to come out of trance . . . That's right . . . Good . . . Okay . . .

I am going to open the discussion up to questions or comments, but feel free to keep anything to yourself you want to keep to yourself, or to share anything you want is fine. It's up to you. Okay. So questions or comments from the peanut gallery?

Member of the audience: There's a question I did not understand.

O'Hanlon: Yeah.

Audience: Maybe I missed something, but how did you know that this was going to be a relationship, possibly with a woman, because I've dealt recently with work relationships that created great anxiety?

O'Hanlon *(to the questioner):* I didn't know. How did you know that?

Audience: Because of some of the evidence . . .

O'Hanlon *(to Stan):* Okay. So we can ask you: Is the person you need to talk to a woman? Is this a relationship thing?

Stan: Yeah.

O'Hanlon: Well, I had a guess about that, I must admit. I didn't know. I had no idea. He didn't tell me; so I don't know. But I did have to guess about it. How? Partly, I had to guess about . . . It was the way he said it at the beginning. It was sort of vague, you know, "I need to talk to this person." And the other thing is that as I told something that had to do with a relationship, he seemed to respond in some way. He smiled. I don't know what. He was giving me some clue . . . See, what I think is that clients teach me. I don't know when I start, and that they teach me as I start . . . with a few vague sort of things that I know about and I can think of, and then he starts to teach me what's important to him by what he responds to. And I'm just giving . . . to me it's like a smorgasbord. I'm saying this, this, this, this or multiple choice questions, and maybe a little better. Like is this relevant for you? Is this relevant for you? Choose A, B, C, D, E, or all of the above. So he seemed to be teaching me what was relevant for him.

Audience: You really don't ask any more questions than you did?

O'Hanlon: No, usually, I mean in a therapy situation, I'll know a bit more. You know, because we'll have a little more time. Altogether we had 45 minutes for me to do some introductory remarks, do a demonstration, and then have a little discussion afterwards; so I was a little more brief than I usually am in terms of asking for information. So I think I would know a lot more, and I probably would know what he had to do. I would ask that question. But I just didn't want to get into things that I didn't think were immediately relevant for what we needed to do.

Audience: Were you in a trance yourself?

O'Hanlon: Yes.

Audience: Were your eyes closed?

O'Hanlon: No, they sometimes go like this. I was watching him essentially the whole time. And that's where my attention was, and that's the kind of trance I went into. If you did a trance with me, I'd have my glasses off, my eyes closed, and I'd be more internally focused. This was an externally focused trance, which is what I do when I teach, and it's the one I do when I do therapy as well. This is a particular kind of one where I just sort of cut you folks out. I noticed it when you went up, and I didn't even notice until you did that there was noise from there. So that is what brought it into my awareness, just as I saw you move; otherwise, I was pretty well in trance.

Audience: Do you ever work interactively on a verbal level with a client?

O'Hanlon: Yes, I do sometimes, and I just didn't have anything particular—again, because I usually am not searching for hidden information or anything like that. There usually isn't anything . . . If they feel moved to talk, though they are welcome to talk to me. In some clients, I develop a sort of style with them where it's much more conversational. With some people, I'll want to talk to them within the trance. What do you need to tell me? Whatever you need to do? That kind of stuff.

In this, I didn't particularly want to know any information. I was just saying, "Go inside and do some stuff, here's some stuff you can do, here are some possibilities." And he was responding to me nonverbally, and I had guesses about whether that was relevant. Sometimes I do a lot more dialogue. Sometimes his eyes are open, and we are looking at each other, too. So that's a different style, too.

Audience: May I hear something from the gentleman about his experience?

Stan: Sure, it was nice. It was interesting in the beginning. He mentioned a lot of words about comfort, I don't know, I just really deepened. Like within a second. It took me a while to get there, but when you said all those words like "comfort," it was kind of interesting. I was just sort of floating around and listening to his words, and it was really humorous toward the end. It's hard for me to . . .

O'Hanlon: Not crack up, huh?

Stan: I maintained that level of trance, I guess. It just felt really good.

There's not . . . my mind was not really active, engaged, or thinking, except in that last minute. I'm sort of talking to myself and saying, "Yeah, this is okay."

O'Hanlon: You see, to me . . . the conversation, we ended it together. He was getting his part of the conversation, which he very . . . definitely could, and you know, gave permission and all that stuff. And he gave me some guidelines, and then he showed me with his behavior that he was coming out of trance, and I said, "Good deal."

Audience: Have you dealt with the issue?

O'Hanlon: I don't know if I dealt with his issue. I would assume that we did somewhat, and gave him some ideas about that, and time will tell whether we deal with the issue in a way that was satisfactory for him. Again, it's like I didn't know that it was about a relationship, about a woman. How in a sense did he . . . within himself? But it could be very helpful and could move him on.

Audience: Will you be seeing him again?

O'Hanlon: No. This is a demonstration. He'll go to his home; I'll go to my home. If he wants to write me a letter, or give me a call, I'd love to hear from him. But would I see him again in my practice?

Audience: If he wants to go on.

O'Hanlon: I would leave it up to him. If he was a client, and he was in my practice, I would leave it up to him. I would say, "What do you think? do you think you want to go out and see how this goes, and see whether you need to come back for another one? Or whether this did it?" I'd leave it up to him.

Audience: Helping this gentleman get into a state of mind that this problem took place and in answering questions, you could assume that that took place during this experience. Do you want to comment on whether you are interested in anything more than that? Is this man going to leave here with a plan of doing or asking? What's the outcome of the induction, other than that?

O'Hanlon: Well, as he says he is satisfied, and he goes out into life, what he does or what he thinks or what he feels is satisfactory to him. I mean that's the ultimate . . . it's customer satisfaction for me. It's the ultimate one. We could have gotten a little more explicit on the goals. But sometimes I get real explicit about how do you know when you are done? How do you know when you get there? And with this, I didn't. I felt that he would know. And I also felt that he was going to *do it*, whether we did the hypnosis or not, he's going to go talk to the person. And that in our conversation that got a little clearer for him both before trance and during it. Would you say that is accurate?

Stan: Yeah.

O'Hanlon: So I didn't feel that I needed to go over a systematic plan with him. I figured he was capable of doing the plan. It's just I wanted to sort of focus him on the memory you need to do this, and he was like, "Oh yeah, I need to do this." That's the sense I got. Yeah?

Audience: A number of times you dwelt on questions like: "How will you know when?"

O'Hanlon: Right.

Audience: What is that?

O'Hanlon: Presupposition. I just implicitly do it. You are creating an image of the future, an idea of the future that there will be a time when that will happen. But now you are just thinking, negotiating. "When will it happen, how will you know it, when will you know it's the truth?"

I just want to say just a few concluding sort of comments; i.e., the kind of hypnosis that I am talking about very much opens up possibilities for people to do things inside; i.e., to think of things differently and to change their physiological processes to change their . . . how they're doing things, make new images of problem-free futures, to go back into the past and get resources and things like that. I'm suggesting the doing, but I'm doing it in a very permissive way, so I am not imposing my idea of what solution should be. But I'm channeling their thinking. Someone once asked me in training, "Well, I know you don't want to put words in your clients' mouths." I said, "That's wrong; I want to put words in their mouths; I want to put thoughts in their minds." More than that, I think, maybe a little more clearly stated, I want to bring forth from them certain thoughts that they wouldn't have thought before they interacted with me. I want to bring forth certain associations and certain emotions, if you will, that they wouldn't have thought. I want to bring forth certain internal and external doings that they wouldn't have done before we had this conversation. And to me, hypnosis is a conversation—not something someone does *to* somebody, but something that we are doing together. And what emerges from that conversation, I think, is what is appropriate for both of us. And he seemed to think that it was appropriate for him; I thought it was appropriate for me, and we were happy about it. Hopefully, we'll have a conversation until we are both happy about how the conversation is going. And then hopefully the conversation will make a difference experientially and in his external life, which he wants to make a difference. So that can be a solution-oriented hypnosis. This is obviously just a brief overview and a brief skimming, but I wanted you to have a sense, to see and hear the practice of it.

Commentary

William Hudson O'Hanlon, M.S.

I'd like to say a few things about solution-oriented hypnosis. A few years ago I went to the Evolution of Psychotherapy Conference and it got me thinking about where therapy has gone, where therapy is going and what it is all about. For me, the evolution of psychotherapy has come down to this: Psychotherapy started out oriented mainly toward discovering the causes and origins of problems. Somewhere in your past the cause of your current disorder happened. It was either genetic, biochemical or developmental. The most prevalent model for most therapists, until recently, was the psychodynamic model, which holds that something happened in your childhood, some trauma or unresolved relationship or psychological issues, that gave rise to current symptoms. In this case, the cure usually consists of having the person sort out what it was that went wrong and fix that, usually in a curative relationship, to solve the problem occurring in the present. Then, in the 1950s, and especially the 1960s and early 1970s, psychotherapy became much more concerned with contemporary, rather than past, causes for problems. With the rise of TA, gestalt, behavioral therapies, family therapy, ego psychology, and other present-oriented techniques and models, the therapist viewed the present symptom or problem as largely a function of present causes or maintenance. These models said, in essence, "Well, past causes rely on a lot of speculations and interpretation, but present causes are much more available for inspection by both client and therapist, so let's focus on those to change the symptom."

After studying with Erickson and being steeped in his way of working for some years, I started to have a different orientation, and I started to notice it in many other people's work. Instead of looking for the causes of peoples' problems, this approach involved more intervention. Instead of searching for explanations, this approach searched for solutions. It was not always future-oriented, but if it dealt with the past, it was with a different slant. Instead of looking for what went wrong with people, it focused on what people did right or what their strengths, abilities and life

74

learnings were that could help them solve their current difficulties. Instead of being oriented toward pathology and explaining why there was a problem, it was oriented toward solutions and possibilities. Erickson once told me that he had no theory of psychotherapy. I don't think that is really true. He had no consistent theory of psychopathology, but he did have a theory of intervention. He had clear and consistent ideas about how to intervene.

In this solution-oriented approach, people are seen as the experts on solving their own problems. They have all the "answers within" (Lankton & Lankton, 1983). The therapist's job is to orient people's attention to these resources and to create the context in which the person can get access to them. There are various ways to do this and I have detailed them in two books (O'Hanlon & Weiner-Davis, 1989; O'Hanlon & Wilk, 1987). For present purposes, we can distinguish between hypnotic and nonhypnotic ways to orient people toward solutions.

The way I decide whether to use an hypnotic approach is to determine whether the presenting problem is of a voluntary/deliberate nature. A voluntary/deliberate problem is one that people could do if asked to do it. For example, if someone asked a therapist to help them stop smoking, they could show the therapist precisely how they smoked. Since they could do this deliberately, this would be considered a voluntary/deliberate problem. In contrast, if a person came to a therapist complaining of migraine headaches and asked for pain control or elimination of the headaches, they almost certainly couldn't show the therapist their headache upon request. This type of problem is what I call involuntary. It's not that people are claiming, "I can't help it." Most people present their therapy problems with a claim that they can't help what they are doing or can't change or stop what they are doing. This distinction is based only on whether or not they could *produce* the symptom upon request.

An involuntary complaint seems to me appropriate for hypnosis. That is, hypnosis seems to be able to affect the stuff we don't usually have a conscious deliberate influence on. Involuntary problems include things that go on inside your bag of bones, your skin, as opposed to behavioral things. So I usually do hypnosis with physiological problems, obsessional thinking, affective issues, self-image issues, memory problems (either flashback or amnesias), etc. Anything that is not usually under your conscious control.

What is different about solution-oriented hypnosis from the traditional hypnotic orientations? Traditional hypnosis usually has one of two goals: to reprogram negative beliefs into more positive ones, or to uncover repressed material. Solution-oriented hypnosis assumes that people already have the ability to change their perceptions, change their attention, go into trance, do all the trance phenomena; that they have the ability, with some stimulation and gentle nudges from the therapist, to discover their own answers to the problems they face.

Indirect techniques, like storytelling, analogies, and interspersed suggestions, are used to invite clients to evoke and apply their previously unused potential and skills to their problems.

The therapist in this approach is not an expert at knowing the answers for the client, only at creating a climate that facilitates such solution making. The therapist doesn't come to the hypnotic encounter knowing what the client should do to solve the problem or burdened down with a lot of theories and explanations. In Zen, there is a saying: In the beginner's mind, there are many possibilities, in the expert's mind, there are few. Solution-oriented hypnosis is a way to approach clients and therapy with a beginner's mind.

While the session presented here is not a wildly successful or profound example of my work, it shows the technique and direction of the work very well. In some ways I'm glad it's not too magical or dramatic, as workshop demonstrations are often so different from everyday sessions. This session is typical of the kind of trancework I do with my clients on a day-to-day basis.

References

Lankton, S., & Lankton, C. (1983). *The answer within: A clinical framework of Ericksonian hypnotherapy.* New York: Brunner/Mazel.

O'Hanlon, B., & Wilk, J. (1987). *Shifting contexts: The generation of effective psychotherapy.* New York: Guilford.

O'Hanlon, W., & Weiner-Davis, M. (1989). *In search of solutions: A new direction in psychotherapy.* New York: Norton.

Commentary

Ernest L. Rossi, Ph.D.

Bill O'Hanlon's demonstration of "solution-oriented hypnosis" illustrates some of the strengths as well as the problems we all share in developing Erickson's permissive hypnotherapeutic approaches. In the most general terms, O'Hanlon's demonstration raises the basic question: How can we generate an optimal balance between randomness and specificity to optimize an ideally creative and therapeutic encounter?

First, let's recognize the strengths of this demonstration. It is hard to argue with success! This subject, Stan, was satisfied with his therapeutic response to O'Hanlon's permissive approach. Stan obviously experienced relief from his initial anxiety when he said toward the end, "It just felt really good. . . . Yeah, this is okay." Stan acknowledged he was aware that O'Hanlon "mentioned a lot of words about comfort," and he was able to respond with good feeling. This is an example of what has been called "indirect associative focusing" (Erickson & Rossi, 1980) to evoke an *ideodynamic* response: The permissive and apparently random stories, words, and behavior of the therapist can activate real mind-body *dynamic* responses within the subject.

The broad range of topics presented by O'Hanlon's indirect associative focusing gave the subject carte blanche to pick up and utilize whatever he could in any way he could. This reminded me of Erickson's "going fishing" approach, in which he would seem to free associate in a casual manner and tell all sorts of stories while the patient was in trance. Erickson was not being casual, however. He was always watching the patient carefully for an involuntary response, a minimal behavioral cue, that indicated he had hit indirectly upon something important for the patient. Erickson was looking ("fishing") for whatever emotional responses he might be tripping off to learn the nature of the patient's problem and dynamics. He was looking for something *specific* in his apparently permissive and *random* indirect approach.

This "going fishing" approach is especially appropriate when seeing for the first time a patient who has a vague complaint such as "anxiety," just as O'Hanlon is doing here in this demonstration. At this initial stage of therapy, however, Erickson *was* looking for sources of problems as well as inner resources for problem resolution.

I believe the audience member who asked the question "Do you ever work interactively on a verbal level with a client?" was hinting at something important that was missing from this demonstration. I need to learn as much as I can about the subject's responses to my words and interventions during hypnosis. Especially in the beginning, I tend to use short permissive hypnotherapeutic "trances" so I can get some immediate verbal feedback from the client that will help me focus my next intervention more specifically for that particular person's problems.

This is a basic problem for all the indirect, permissive approaches of hypnotherapy. How do we get adequate feedback about the appropriateness of our intervention? This is the main reason I have spent much of my exploratory efforts in the past few years learning more about ideodynamic signaling (Rossi & Cheek, 1988). Learning to recognize a patient's involuntary minimal cues and ideodynamic signals allows therapists to introduce much needed specificity to balance the randomness of the nondirective, permissive approach.

We urgently need a deeper theoretical rationale for the relationship between the use of *random* free associations, stories and metaphors in all forms of psychotherapy and *specificity* in responding appropriately to the patient's communications. I am currently exploring a new mathematical development that may be applied to optimizing the ideal balance of randomness and specificity to facilitate creativity in the human encounter. This new development is called "chaos theory."

In brief, a revolution is currently taking place in physics (Davies, 1989), biology, and psychology (Rossi, 1989a, 1989b) in applying nonlinear dynamics to understanding all forms of deterministic but highly complex and essentially nonpredictable forms of behavior, information, and communication. This paradigm can provide a theoretical foundation for understanding the optimal balance between random free associations and specific communications and directives in facilitating the evolution of more effective patterns of behavior and consciousness. It is an exciting new direction, as we break with the past in a search for a better future in our present.

References

Davies, P. (1989). *The new physics.* New York: Cambridge University Press.
Erickson, M., & Rossi, E. (1980). The indirect forms of suggestion. In E. Rossi (Ed.), *The collected works of Milton H. Erickson on hypnosis. Vol. 1. The nature of hypnosis and suggestion.* New York: Irvington.

Rossi, E. (1989a). Archetypes as strange attractors. *Psychological Perspectives, 21*(1), 4–14.

Rossi, E. (1989b). Chaos, determinism, and free will. *Psychological Perspectives, 21*(1), 110–127.

Rossi, E., & Cheek, D. (1988). *Mind-body therapy: Ideodynamic healing in hypnosis.* New York: Norton.

Facilitating "Creative Moments" in Hypnotherapy

Ernest L. Rossi, Ph.D.

Rossi: We are here to learn about "creative moments" and three indirect forms of suggestion. What are creative moments? I feel they are the essence of all forms of psychotherapy. They are moments when we have an "ah-ha" experience. These are the moments that are celebrated in all the literature of consciousness—from the satori of zen to the mystical moments of communion with God for mystics. In our work we settle for more humble insights.

The first clue that a creative moment is taking place is so common that it almost seems ridiculous to talk about it: It is the moment when a person pauses. You know, you're talking, then the client pauses, and they look off. That's the moment for the therapist to shut up. Sometimes I'll shut up in mid-sentence. I'll start saying something, and the person looks off, abstract, and boom, I'll stop just like that. And the client never seems to notice that I've stopped, because they are so busy inside. And, of course, that's where we want people to be.

How do we facilitate those creative moments? That was the essence of what I was trying to develop in *Dreams and the Growth of Personality* (Rossi, 1972/1985). When I later met Milton H. Erickson, this was the basis of my connection with him. I wasn't so much interested in hypnosis, but in how hypnosis could be used to access a person's creativity. I believe the essence of my work with Erickson was simply to outline all the indirect forms of suggestion that he was using. Those all appear in Volume I of the *Collected Papers* (1980a). If I had to do it over again, I would not call them "indirect forms of suggestion." I now like

Transcript of a demonstration given in Phoenix, December 1985.

to call them the "language of human facilitation," because "suggestion" is a misnomer. The concept of suggestion might have been important 200 years ago, but now it is death. It is death to the therapist.

Hypnosis is not suggestion; it's not influence communication' it's not prestige; it's not covert conditioning. Those ideas all lead to the death of the therapist, because suggestion unfortunately does work once in a while, and that acts as an intermittent reinforcer for the therapist. After a while the therapist really thinks there's magic in his words or his points of view, and he stops thinking creatively about the client. The therapist gets more and more narcissistic on how he is going to suggest this or that to program the patient. That is death for the psychotherapist! Satan get thee from my door! That's the corrupter of the creativity of the therapist.

What then is the "language of human facilitation"? It's all these approaches to helping a person turn inward to access their own resources. This morning I tried to describe how the state-dependent memory and learning systems (Rossi, 1986) help a person to access the psychophysiological locus of a problem, to access the places where their learning stopped, and to access the inner resources that can reevoke the learning that can resolve the problem they're struggling with.

I'm going to outline three of these means of facilitating creative moments—what used to be called "indirect suggestion," now called the "language of human facilitation"—and then I am going to ask for a few volunteers. But since I am very much interested in integrating my early work on dreams and the expansion of awareness with my more recent work with Erickson, I am going to ask for volunteers who may have had a dream about this congress. In that way, we might also get a message from the unconscious that is relevant to all of us. So there are a number of levels on which I'd like to operate this afternoon. I'd like to work with two or three people, if possible—not very long, perhaps not more than 5 or 10 minutes each, because I hope to demonstrate a variety of approaches. Yet that does not mean that this is merely a demonstration. Some of the most interesting talks I've had with Carl Rogers lately are precisely about this format of working, what he calls "demonstration therapy." He has letters from people going back 25, 30 years ago, when he saw them only for 5 or 10 minutes—or maybe 20 minutes—for a demonstration on stage. Apparently, there is a heightening of consciousness. A person who has the guts to come up here is activating all their sensory perceptual memory systems. Gunnison (1985) recently pointed out these unrecognized connections between hypnosis in the sense of accessing and reframing inner processes and the process of Rogerian counseling. So that is what we're doing; we are always accessing. We are always utilizing the inner resources of the client.

There are three approaches you are going to be seeing me use over and over again: the first is simply asking questions that the conscious mind cannot answer. Think about that for a moment. Usually, when we ask questions, we want an answer. Not so with the language of human facilitation. We ask questions to access inner resources, to access different states of being. Maybe human consciousness itself evolved when the protohuman invented the semantic form we call "the question," because the question is a device that causes us to do inner work. So when I ask someone, "What part of your body is feeling most comfortable right now?" What a surprising question! To answer that question a person—what does this person have to do? They have to go inside; they have to tune into themselves. That's what I want them to do. That's beginning the process of accessing inner resources to facilitate a creative moment.

Another aspect of the language of human facilitation I'm sure all of you use, is what we popularly call "channeling" [or "information transduction" as I would prefer to call it today]. Those shifts from words to emotions to imagery to cognitions, etc. I'll show you some special approaches that I am developing that came out of my work with Erickson: having a person channel a feeling that perhaps cannot be expressed in any other way, for example, through a kinesthetic movement of their hand, their arm. In general, whenever I ask a person, "Let your hands do such and such," or "Let your fingers do such and such," or "Let your eyelids do such and such," you know I am using this process of channeling. I'm helping a person switch sensory-perceptual modalities within to help them access more adequately their own creative resources.

The third approach is what I've called the "implied directive," which is very closely related to what has been called the "conscious-unconscious double bind." Today I prefer to call them "therapeutic binds" (Rossi & Ryan, in press). Whenever you hear me say to someone, "If your unconscious is willing to deal with such and such problem, your eyelids might do such and such" [e.g., close] or "If your unconscious has done such and such inner work then your head will do such and such involuntary response" [e.g., nodding], that's really the form of the implied directive. I'm giving a directive, but the carrying out of the directive is really placed within the person. Again, I'm accessing inner resources [and asking the unconscious to signal with an observable involuntary response when the inner process is carried through].

Something you might see me do is the typical double-bind, the therapeutic bind, that goes something like, "If it's really okay for your unconscious to review the sources of that problem, you'll find your eyelids starting to close. You'll find yourself getting more comfortable. But if there's another issue that needs to be discussed first, you'll find yourself getting a little bit antsy; you'll find yourself getting a little bit restless, until that new issue comes up clearly in your mind." So, you see, whatever choice a person makes, it is a move in a therapeutic direction. I don't presume to know what issue a person needs to deal with. I let their unconscious decide it. If their unconscious says, "This is the issue," they'll find themselves getting quieter, because that's the way nature works. When we are really doing inner work, we are not moving our hands, our legs; we are kind of fixed. These are the everyday catalepsies (Erickson & Rossi, 1981). But when we are doing inner work, and we are struggling to get something out sometimes, then there's tension in us, then we may snap our fingers [shift our posture, etc.]. So we utilize these natural mental mechanisms. Again, we are not suggesting, we are utilizing naturistic processes.

I wonder if we have anyone in the audience who has had a recent dream, hopefully a short one, that they would like to share with us and work with for a few minutes. If there are two or three of you, please come up and have a seat on the stage, and I'll work with each of you in turn. At least two or three of you.

(People are walking to the stage and there is some conversation in getting them settled on the stage—about microphones, etc.)

Gloria

Rossi: Can you share a dream with us?

Gloria: I would like to. I hadn't thought about it being about this conference until you asked. The night before I left New York to come, I had a beautiful dream about my son's little hamster giving birth to seven babies. And it was a very sweet dream and it was very special, and I mentioned that to my son that morning before I took the plane to come to Phoenix. And when I called that night to check in, I learned that the hamster had indeed given birth to seven babies that afternoon. And I thought that was about my own family, and something that was going on there. But when you asked the question, I was sure it was about this conference.

Rossi: Thank you. That's very beautiful. And as I look at you, I can notice the sclera of your eyes getting red. You're really feeling touched by the impact of your own dream. That's right. So *if it really will be okay for you to tune inward and really receive something more about that dream, you'll find,* that's right, that's right. That's it, experiencing that deepening comfort. That's it, the *eyelids beginning to blink,* that's right. And if there really is so much more, that's it, that's right. If there really is so much more of . . . *those eyes can eventually close, as the memories, your son, hamster, and seven babies.* That's right. That's right. Hmm-uh. And that's it . . . continuing to receive . . . That's right, that's right.

And now she's manifesting a characteristic vibratory motion of the eyelids, which has been mentioned in hypnotic literature for over 200 years as one of the indicators of a person going into a hypnotic trance. Others, including Erickson, felt that that was an indicator of very intense inner work being done. That's right. And there's a slight pulling together of the forehead, a slight frowning—all indications that some intense work is being done at this time. Hypnosis is not passivity; it is really relevant [intense inner work]. Yes. The nose is beginning to get slightly reddened as the autonomic nervous system shifts are taking place, facial dilation. There's a whole series of psychophysiological changes. And as I look at her hands, I notice that's her left that's on top of her right, suggesting that this woman has possibly quite a bit of right hemispheric dominance. You notice that her head is also tilted to the right. That causes a shift in nasal breathing, that also causes a reflexive change in cerebral hemispheric dominance toward the right hemisphere (Rossi, 1986). A lot of people feel that hypnosis is accessing right hemisphericity. I feel that's too simple, though this client is certainly manifesting that in a classical way. And if that is really going well, that's it. Already I can see that her response to my question, there was a minimal movement of a head, "Yes." I didn't even have to ask her. I was about to suggest that if it was going well, her unconscious could nod her head "yes." But her unconscious did it even before. See what's happening. I'm picking up all these minimal cues; there's a conversation going on between us in a nonverbal way. That's right. That's right. *And if it will be okay, in another moment or two, for those eyes to open, for you to share just one or two things, one or two things that could be shared publicly, and allowing all the rest to remain within the unconscious where it can continue its creative work. If that's really okay, those fingers will begin to move; your hands you'll stretch; and finally open your eyes coming alert, awake and refreshed. Hi!*

Gloria: I didn't want to come back. I was very relaxed.

Rossi: See, there is a reluctance to actually move her fingers and follow my directive. Would you say you are completely awake at this time?

Gloria: I think so.

Rossi: Okay. The realities of the situation unfortunately do require you to come fully awake, but you can take some of this in your own everyday life. And I'm going to tell you in a moment just how to do it, after you've shared just one or two things with us that're okay to share.

Gloria: I felt that my dream was symbolic of the fertileness that will be here, and the rebirth of learning, and also symbolic of some rebirth that I am going through personally.

Rossi: Okay, thank you. And now, I'd like to give you that hint about how you can do this inner work by yourself. You are just a genius of inner accessing. You are beautiful. I want to thank you for allowing me to work with you.

Are you aware of the ultradian rhythms in everyday life? Okay. This was the subject of one of my papers (Rossi, 1986), where I point out the connections between the ultradian rhythms and the common everyday trance, meditation, and inner work. In short, all of us go through a natural psychobiological rhythm every hour and a half. At night we dream every hour and a half. Even during the daytime, this hour and a half cycle continues. Our society recognizes it. We go to work at 9:00 a.m., an hour and a half later coffee break time, an hour and half after that, lunch time, and so on throughout the day. A lot of research has shown that when people don't let themselves have that natural rest cycle, that's the source of the disruption in psychobiological rhythms and a source of psychosomatic illness.

I found personally that when I really tune into my body and I let myself close my eyes and go into—some might call it inner work, some might call it meditation, some might call it trance—I simply say to myself, "I'm going to let the unconscious do what it needs to do." And I "go out" for about 15 or 20 minutes. In other words, that's the natural psychobiological rhythm for doing inner work. And if I have a particular issue that I want to deal with, I'll ask myself, "Will my unconscious deal with this issue? And will I know the answer in five minutes? Tomorrow? Next week?"

In other words, it's very open ended. So I'd strongly recommend to you that you really allow yourself to use those natural rhythms to facilitate your own inner work and this creative process that you sense is going on in you. And, of course, you can't always do it, if you're driving along on the freeway and your ultradian rest comes up, you can't suddenly go out, but you can be aware that it is there and use it to become hyperalert, say, be even more aware of traffic. Use it as a kind of hyperalert trance. In other words, it's a way of working with yourself every day to facilitate the inner work. Okay? Thank you.

I really tried to put a lot in that. I think that's a message I have for all of you about really tuning into our psychobiology. In my dream book, the second edition that has just come out (Rossi, 1972/1985), I talk about some of my own really profound experiences during the ultradian rhythms. For many years when I worked with Milton, we would quit work usually around 3:00 or 4:00 in the afternoon. I'd wheel him into the house, and I'd go back out to the study. I would lie on the couch and I would go into self-hypnosis. Of course, I'm sure the old fox, was seeding a lot of my so-called objective work with him with personal suggestions. But it was during those ultradian self-hypnotic periods that I was able to experience visual hallucinations, mystical states of consciousness—what in the historical literature has been called lucid somnambulism, i.e., getting into a state within yourself where suddenly you realize you're in a dream state, but you're conscious. And you can start working with all of your own memory systems. After being an analyst for about 20 years, I was able to access memories that had never come clearer to me before. So this is a very very powerful approach that becomes powerful in direct proportion to your increasing sensitivity to yourself. In this sense, it is a fail-safe approach. Because if you are not sensitive to yourself, you can't get access, and if you are not sensitive to yourself, of course, you would only mess yourself up [so it's best not to get access]. That's a kind of a bonus of the approach. It has taken me many years to get to this level of sensitivity, and I still can't call it up that well, but enough to keep me working at it. Do we have another subject?

Sally

Sally: I woke up this morning in the middle of this dream when we got our wake-up call. The dream was just going on . . . And in the dream, I was at The Conference of the Evolution of Psychotherapy, but it was in Mexico. And our hotel room was at the top of this high, high summit. And the room was at the top of this tall, tall pole, and it was like balancing precariously on the pole. And it was very frightening, but it was a magnificent view. And so, there was this mixture of fear and just awe and excitement. And then during the day we went to the conference, but the conference was climbing the steep summit—this mountain. And there was a man that was helping us climb this very steep dangerous cliff. And we got to the top, there was a flood of water. I didn't know that it was raining at the time. And people were being washed off the cliff and were having to hold . . . not to be washed away. And that was about the time when my wake-up call came, so I don't know how it turned out.

Rossi: Wow! That does sound like a big dream to me. Do you have any conscious impressions of it?

Sally: I haven't really had time to play with it very much. It felt like there was some expectations of some very important things happening, as a result of this conference. And certainly there are a lot of very new important things happening in my life right now, and precarious.

Rossi: What about the Mexican part?

Sally: That's definitely a part of it. I'm just recently separated, so it was a real new period of my life.

Rossi: Are you of Mexican descent?

Sally: No, but I was an Indian in another life. And it was an Indian that was helping us. Okay, I said I was an Indian in another life, and it was an Indian that was helping us up the mountain.

Rossi: Hm-hm. There were two high places. There was the high tower, as well as the high mountain, and both of them were a little dangerous being up there. Do you have any conscious awareness of what that danger could be?

Sally: Not really. I think the danger is the fear of reaching new places that I've not experienced before, and it feels that I'm at a point where that's just about to happen—and it's scary.

Rossi: The fear of reaching new places, places that you've never been before, and you can feel that's about to happen, and it is happening. Can you feel what's happening in your face right now?

Sally: Yes.

Rossi: Are you willing to share it?

Sally: I don't know if I can put words to it.

Rossi: Could I put some words to it? There's just a curious vibration in your right cheek. Is that what you've experienced? Do you know what that is? [A small tic-like movement of her right cheek that unfortunately was not picked up by the video camera.]

Sally: No.

Rossi: Whatever it is, it's trying to tell us something.

Sally: *(she laughs)*

Rossi: Have you ever experienced hypnosis? Would you like to experience an interesting kind of hypnotic induction? *(long pause as Rossi moves his hand slowly toward hers and she watches obviously fascinated)* And will it be okay for me to guide that hand upward?*(long pause as Rossi makes some slight but confusing movements over her hands until one of her hands starts to move involuntarily up toward his)* That's right. That's right. That's right. And already all signs of that vibration in the cheek are gone as we channel the energy in this new way. That's right. Really experiencing the comfort of allowing that to continue just that way. And *if it will really be okay . . . for you to receive something, you'll find that comfort deepening, and your eyes closing.* That's right. And really receiving, that's right, that's right. And *as you continue to receive, your hand will begin drifting downward very slowly as you receive the memories, courage, understandings, that's right.* That's right. Simply receiving. That's right. That's right. *So by the time that hand comes to rest in your lap, you will know just one or two things of what you receive that you can share with us.* That's right. *Just one or two things that can truly help you.* That's right. That's right. That's it. That's it. *Taking just another moment to complete that work, so that you really really know.* That's right. That's it. Hm-uh. Very fine. Hi! How are you doing?

Sally: Fine. That's incredible! When you first put your hand there, before you even said anything, I felt my hand starting to be pulled up.

Rossi: Do you want to say something more about how that hand got pulled up?

Sally: Yes, it felt like a magnet drawing my hand up. I could really feel the energy just . . . it felt magnetic.

Rossi: Were you lifting the hand, or was it going by itself?

Sally: It was just being pulled.

Rossi: You did not have voluntary control?

Sally: I wasn't consciously lifting it.

Rossi: So this is an indication that an autonomous process was activated. She experienced it as a magnet pulling her hand up. And, of course, dear old Mesmer, 200 years ago, used magnets because the metaphor of the magnet is associated with something happening on an involuntary autonomous level. So it's as if her hand was moving by itself, drawn by a magnet. And it's that involuntary quality that's a classical characteristic of hypnosis. That's a classical way of saying, "Hey, we really accessed something—we've accessed the unconscious within—so that we are getting closer to what we need to. Can you share one or two things with us of what you received from within?

Sally: I just had one thought. I just kept hearing the same thing over and over again—that *it's time to take the climb.*

Rossi: Over and over again, it's time to take the climb. And you really feel that, don't you? Yes. It's like . . . *(he takes a deep breath)* And this is a decision you're making. This one's for you! Thank you very much.

Fay

Rossi: Hi!

Fay: My name is Fay.

Rossi: Hi, Fay. *(he takes several deep breaths)* Ready to share a dream?

Fay: I dreamed last night that I was standing out in front of the conference building—it's very short. There is someone else with me. I don't know who—a wise man. And we're looking at the sky, and the sky is all lit in either pastel yellow or gold or, or pink. And the message was to me: "You need to use the pink."

Rossi: The message was "You need to use the pink." Wow!

Fay: The pink light.

Rossi: The pink what?

Fay: The pink light.

(Laughter, whistles)

Rossi: I think we all like that. Is it funny?

Fay: No, no.

Rossi: I'm sorry. I'm not thinking it's funny so much as I'm delighted by the . . . Yes?

Fay: It seems spiritual, it seems feminine, it seems those kinds of things.

Rossi: Yes.

Fay: I understand now. You were whistling, you with me, you were laughing with me because it is a good dream.

Rossi: Yes, I sure think so. *(he takes several deep breaths)* Are you feeling . . . ?

Fay: I'm feeling more relaxed, yes.

Rossi: Do you have any conscious idea about that thing?

Fay: Only what I told you—that it seems spiritual, it seems feminine. That's what it seems.

Rossi: Spiritual and feminine. Truly.

Fay: Feminine meaning being softer.

Rossi: Softer. *Can you experience softness within yourself right now?* A little hard?

Fay: It's vulnerable.

Rossi: It's vulnerable. That's right. Just continue. That's it. Very fine. And her eyes have closed now, after *she did a momentary eye fixation all by herself.* And really continuing now—oh, that's it. That's right. That's right. Yes. The spiritual, the feminine, that pink light in the sky. *(long pause)* That's right. Hm-uh. And a moment ago there was a deeper, slower roll of both eyelids, suggesting another shift of unconsciousness to a slightly deeper level. That's right. That's right. And it's very obvious how her whole system is kind of relaxed now as she focuses on the inner work. *(long pause)* That's right. That's right. Exactly that! That's it. That's right. That's right—*seizing, really seizing that! That's right, and a slight little nod of her head,* "Yes," to let me know that she is in touch with me. She did seize that. That's right. Hi. Take another moment or two. That's right. That's it. And you can really feel the depth of that emotion, and yet another part of you can watch it objectively— simply receiving. Experiencing. That's it. *And you can experience those tears and yet really receive what's coming with them.* That's it. Staying with that for another moment. *Receiving the message of those tears.* That's right. Hm-uh. That's it. And I say the relaxing of that is as I see her give a sigh of relaxation. That's right. Taking another moment now simply to pull it all together, knowing that this inner work is going to continue entirely on its own. It's going to continue in your dreams, it's going to continue in your relations with others; it's going to continue in the depth of your developing spiritual insights, and the reclaiming of all that lost feminine. That's right. Just one or two things that can be shared publicly. Hi!

Fay: I'm not quite back yet. I feel very soft. I feel—I'm not quite back yet. I feel very soft. What hit first was, "Let go of fear." *"Let go of fear."*

Rossi: Let go of fear, is what came to you first?

Fay: And it generalized. It generalized from letting go of fear inside of me to working with people in therapy for that to be a crucial thing to everybody here. I kept seeing the outside of the building. All right. Then I got, "Let go of competition." And the last is that I'm working on my body—I'm giving up smoking—and of getting my body in good condition again. And it kept saying, "Love to go soft. Don't demand to go soft and love yourself. The more you love yourself, the more you can give it up."

Rossi: Thank you for that. I would like to just share with you that I am very much in the same place. It ain't easy to be 52.

Fay: It's real hard to be vulnerable.

Rossi: Yes. the approach I am using with myself—that ultradian approach—is the most healing approach I have found. Several times a day to really let myself go into comfort, or to say, letting go, going into the softness. That's the parasympathetic system—that's exactly what we both need for that kind of inner healing. To allow the energy to go within so the creative work can facilitate itself. And we need to do that every day. We need to cherish ourselves. And as we enrich ourselves, only then can we come out and enrich others. That's what our work is all about.

Fay: Thank you so much.

Rossi: Thank you, too.

Janet

Rossi: Hi!

Janet: Hello.

Rossi: Do you have a dream?

Janet: My dream happened last week. The dream was as follows: I was seated in a chair, a very comfortable easy chair.

Rossi: You were seated in a very comfortable easy chair.

Janet: In front of me was a man seated in the same type of a chair, and he was a hypnotist. *(laughter)* His face was not very clear to me, but I remembered that his eyes were set wide apart, and he seemed to have a very gentle and compassionate face. And, we were working, I guess, and all of a sudden myself and the chair took off. And, you know, when you are driving your car, and you can see a straight road, it goes to a point of infinity, and the lines come this way. Well for me, it was the opposite. The lines were wide here, and my chair took off into infinity to a point so I could see the lines that I came from. Do you see the picture?

Rossi: In other words, you were going backward into infinity—into the flight of infinity, but there was wide area in front of you?

Janet: Yes. And when I got very, very, very far away, I knew there was still room to go further, but I was already at a point. I said, "This is not the time." And my chair, with me, came back. And as I came back, and the chair plopped itself in front of the hypnotist, I walk out. And it was an ideal feeling about my dream. It was a very comfortable dream that I had a choice of when I could do work. And, you see, the dream happened to me last week when I was in Germany, so it's almost like I wanted to do some work when I had some resources for myself.

Rossi: You wanted to do some work to access resources for yourself?

Janet: No. At a time when I had resources to myself, and while I was in Germany last week, I felt it was not the time to deal with something the dream was bringing to me. And so I chose—this is how I look at it—that I chose to wake up and literally come back in my chair into the here and now.

Rossi: The here and now, which is now. Wow, that is really profound.

Janet: When you asked the question, "Did anyone have a dream about this conference?" Well, at first I was stunned because it was the first moment that I realized that maybe the dream had something to do with this conference. I had not though about it.

Rossi: Wow! I very much enjoy looking at your eyes. Notice how we have similar color eyes. Isn't it rather remarkable? You have green eyes, do you not?

Janet: Yes.

Rossi: And so do I.

Janet: Yours are a little more bluish.

Rossi: They might be changing now. I could tell you many stories about my green eyes, but I won't. Have you ever experienced hypnosis?

Janet: I have here in Phoenix at a very small workshop done by the Erickson Foundation last spring. So I have done it once.

Rossi: Would you allow me . . . Would you like to experience a new technique of hypnotic induction?

Place your hands up about like so—a little bit closer together. That's right. And focus on your hands. *And let's pretend for a moment your hands are like magnets, but don't let them move together yet.* You're feeling it already, but don't let them move too much yet, because we want to use this. Because the unconscious is the same way. *When the unconscious wants to say yes, it usually moves people or things together. When the unconscious wants to say no, it usually pushes people or things apart.* That's it. And it's a struggle to keep your eyes open, but keep them open for just a moment. And *if your unconscious wants to say yes to this question, you'll find those hands coming together.* That's it. *Otherwise, you'll find them moving apart.* That's it. And if it will be okay, here and now today to really—that's it—really experience that movement. That's right. And *there's an index finger showing extra movements which suggest to me that that's an ideomotor response of her signaling "yes," it can let me know by moving that finger again. That's right.* Very fine, very fine. And if it will be okay *as this continues, we need to go back only momentarily into infinity.* That's right, *only momentarily, moving into that point of infinity.* That's right. And *making a fast grab at something.* That's it. *Grabbing something, grabbing something that you can bring back very quickly.* that's right. That's it. That's right. Hm-uh. That's it. That's right. Something . . . hm-uh. That's right. Just one or two things, knowing that all the rest will continue all by itself. That's right. That's it. *As soon as those fingers touch, you'll feel it like a bubble popping, popping suddenly coming awake, even though you really don't want to.* Letting yourself suddenly pop awake. That's it. That's it. Uncomfortable. That's it, and yet knowing that we've used up all our time. That's it. That's it, *taking a deeper breath and coming fully awake as those hands touch your thigh.*

Janet: I thought I lost contact with you at one point.

Rossi: What's that?

Janet: I thought I lost contact with you. I don't know.

Rossi: I see.

Janet: I was totally unaware of what you were saying.

Rossi: She totally lost contact with me and was unaware of what I was saying. That is, she truly went into a very profound trance in that very short time.

Janet: I'm curious. What did you say?

Rossi: Of course, this is also the phenomenon of hypnotic amnesia. We really have to stop. And I would like—if you have any doubt about what I am about to say, to read the papers on hypnotic amnesia in volume II of Milton's *Collected Papers* (1980b). The very great value of experiencing hypnotic amnesia, and not allowing the therapist to break in and tell you what was said, that hypnotic amnesia is protecting your unconscious. It's still too vulnerable; it needs to do the work entirely in private. Thank you very much.

Janet: Thank you very much.

References

Erickson, M. (1980a). Notes on minimal cues in vocal dynamics and memory. In E. Rossi (Ed.), *The collected papers of Milton H. Erickson. Vol. I. The nature of hypnosis and suggestion* (pp. 373–377). New York: Irvington.

Erickson, M. H. (1980b). *The collected papers of Milton H. Erickson on hypnosis, Vol. II, Hypnotic alteration of sensory, perceptual and psychophysiological processes* (E. L. Rossi, Ed.). New York: Irvington.

Erickson, M., & Rossi, E. (1981). *Experiencing hypnosis: Therapeutic approaches to altered states.* New York: Irvington.

Gunnison, H. (1985). The uniqueness of similarities: Parallels of Milton H. Erickson and Carl Rogers. *Journal of Counseling and Development, 63,* 561–564.

Rossi, E. (1972/1985). *Dreams and the growth of personality.* New York: Brunner/Mazel.

Rossi, E. (1982). Hypnosis and ultradian cycles: A new state(s) theory of hypnosis? *Journal of Clinical Hypnosis, 25*(1), 21–32.

Rossi, E. (1986). Altered states of consciousness in everyday life: The ultradian rhythms. In B. Wolman (Ed.), *Handbook of altered states of consciousness* (pp. 97–132). New York: Van Nostrand.

Rossi, E., & Ryan, M. (in press). *Creative choice in hypnosis. Vol. IV. The seminars, workshops, and lectures of Milton H. Erickson.* New York: Irvington.

Commentary

Ernest L. Rossi, Ph.D.

This demonstration of a client-centered Ericksonian approach to *facilitating creative moments in hypnotherapy*, with four volunteers whom I had not met previously, illustrates well my typical way of working. Since this was a teaching demonstration, I begin with a general discussion of how I am currently developing Erickson's naturalistic utilization approach to psychotherapy.

I overdramatize a bit to make my first point when I say, "Suggestion is the death of the psychotherapist." But there has been a cruel misunderstanding of my early work with Erickson! Many people, researchers included (Lynn et al., 1988; Stone & Lundy, 1985), have misinterpreted our use of "indirect suggestion" as just another, sneakier way of controlling, manipulating, and programming people. They continue to ignore the open-ended, permissive spirit of our work which has been emphasized again and again. Here are two examples from *Hypnotherapy: An Exploratory Casebook* (Erickson & Rossi, 1979):

> It may be of value for the reader to recognize that an "attitude" or "approach" is being presented with this material rather than a "technique" that is designed to achieve definite and predictable (though limited) results. *The indirect forms of suggestion are most useful for exploring potentialities and facilitating a patient's natural response tendencies rather than imposing control over behavior.* (p. 19)

> Rossi: You emphasize the separation of conscious and unconscious to make sure she leaves it to the unconscious rather than try to work on it with the more limited means of her conscious processes. That is the essence of your hypnotic approach: *depotentiating the conscious mind's limited means and reinforcing unconscious processes with their greater potentialities.*
>
> Erickson: Yes, and the separation is stated in such a way that it has to be accepted because what I'm saying is true.

Rossi: Hypnosis is not a means of directly programming people to do things in one way. With billions of neurological connections in the mind, it is terribly presumptuous to try to program people.

Erickson: It is a very uninformed way.

Rossi: We are allowing the infinite diversity of the unconscious to come forth rather than trying to program one idiotic idea or point of view we may have. There are infinite patterns of learning and ways of doing things. Our approach helps people unlearn their learned limitations. (p. 288)

It is true, as others have emphasized, that Erickson often was manipulative—particularly during his earlier years when he was exploring the nature of suggestion experimentally in the laboratory. In these demonstrations, however, I illustrate Erickson's mature hypno*therapeutic* approach by using three indirect forms of suggestion (which I now prefer to term the "language of human facilitation") to help the volunteers access their own internal realities and actualize their own inner resources for creating a more meaningful and healing way of being (Erickson & Rossi, 1989; Erickson et al., 1976; Rossi, 1986).

Three of the most useful linguistic forms of human facilitation I use in these demonstrations are:

1. *Questions the conscious mind cannot answer* unless the subject turns inward (where we want the subject to do self-exploration);
2. *Information transduction* (called "channeling" in the session) from one modality to another (emotions to imagery and cognitions, and vice versa) to access inner resources;
3. *The general accessing and utilization approach* (called the "implied directive" in the session), which is usually associated with a therapeutic double-bind.

A complete three-step outline that I use for integrating all three of these approaches to 1) initiate therapeutic work ("hypnotic induction"), 2) access and resolve problems, and 3) ratify problem solving is presented elsewhere (Rossi & Cheek, 1988).

A few comments on each of the four volunteers:

Gloria

After she recounts her dream I initiate therapeutic hypnosis with the implied directive (that I now prefer to call the "general accessing and utilization approach") somewhat as follows: "If it really will be okay for you to tune inward and really receive something more about that dream, you will find . . . your eyelids beginning to blink . . . those eyes can eventually close as the memories . . ." That is, eye closure is made contingent on her actually doing some inner work relevant to learning more about her dream.

After a period of facilitating her inner work in a completely nondirective manner, I awaken her with the same general accessing and utilization approach when I say: "And if it will be okay, in another moment or two, for those eyes to open . . . awake and refreshed."

She appears reluctant to awaken (because, after all, this really is too brief a therapeutic trance—most people like to spend at least 15 to 20 minutes in a natural ultradian trance), but she does respond appropriately to the posthypnotic suggestion to say "one or two things that could be shared publicly, and *allowing all the rest to remain within the unconscious* [a naturalistic indirect suggestion for amnesia] where it can continue its creative work . . ."

Sally

It really was a bit of a shock for me to witness that unusual tic suddenly appearing on the subject's right cheek. Obviously, it was a manifestation of the tension she was experiencing on stage in front of about 1000 people. But I also hypothesized that it could be a signal from her unconscious that some important inner process was ready to be accessed and worked with. Nonetheless, I was concerned about the possibility of precipitating a negative therapeutic reaction (it certainly would not be nice for her to be left with a tic in response to our demonstration), so I used a rather subtle but fascinating hypnotic induction I saw Erickson use on a number of occasions when he felt he needed a potent nonverbal approach to distracting the patient from a negative behavior pattern to refocus attention on something more constructive. Her later description of experiencing a *nonvoluntary movement of her hand* to follow mine upward as if it was being pulled by a magnetic force is interesting in the context of the history of hypnosis.

Having safely distracted and transduced her involuntary tic-like kinesthetic cheek response into an involuntary kinesthetic hand levitation, I then proceeded with my customary general accessing and utilization formula: "If it will be really okay for you to receive something, you will find that comfort deepening and your eyes closing."

I use the same verbal formula two more times in quick succession (italicized in the transcript) to rapidly help her access something she needed to know about her dream. She later reports that she did, in fact, receive something she needed to know for her current development: *"It's time to take the climb."*

Fay

My induction here began by first taking a few deep breaths myself to serve as a nonverbal model for her, as well as to relax myself after just narrowly averting a serious misunderstanding (after a moment's reflection, she correctly realized that I was laughing with her, not at her).

The second step in the induction was asking her a question she could only answer by going within: "Can you experience softness within yourself right now?"

Of course, this utilized the exact word *softness* that she had just used with me. Obviously, it was something desirable for her, so I immediately utilized it as an inner-directed, trance-facilitating question.

I was reading her minimal facial cues of suddenly focused inner attention, which I reinforced with "seizing, really seizing that," and she responded with a positive nod of her head. As tears began to flow, I acknowledged them and facilitated information transduction—the shift from emotions to a cognitive awareness—with "receiving the messages of those tears." She did in fact get an important message: "Let go of fear." Since she talked about her role as a therapist, I concluded with a few collegial self-disclosures that could reinforce her need to heal herself. The implied message was "We are all in this together."

Janet

I used my favorite hand kinesthetic general accessing and utilization approach (see Chapter 3 in Rossi & Cheek, 1988) to facilitate trance. Since she manifested a strong, spontaneous involuntary finger movement, I converted it into finger signals when I said, "There's an index finger . . . moving that finger again." Notice how I did not suggest it directly—rather I used the implied directive again!

Unfortunately the video camera was focused entirely on the subject, so it did not record how, when her eyes closed, I purposely turned slowly away from her and cupped my hands over my mouth to "throw my voice" in back of me as far away from her as possible. I hoped that this subtle shift in my voice locus (Erickson, 1980) might give her unconscious the illusion that she was once more moving backward as in her dream to that point of infinity (of her past?) where there apparently was something important for her to receive and/or do (so I suggested "grabbing something that you can bring back very quickly").

When she awakened from this brief trance, she indicated some experience of an altered state when she said, "I lost contact with you at one point." It is hard to believe that she was so far "out" in such a brief trance that she did not receive at least something of what I said on some level. I therefore took it as a working assumption that she actually experienced a hypnotic amnesia as an appropriate protection in this exposed public demonstration. Her apparent hypnotic amnesia strongly suggested to me that she was not ready to talk about her experience, so I ended by emphasizing her need to continue the work in private.

References

Erickson, M. (1980). Notes on minimal cues in vocal dynamics and memory. In E. Rossi (Ed.), *The collected papers of Milton H. Erickson. Vol. I. The nature of hypnosis and suggestion* (pp. 373–377). New York: Irvington.

Erickson, M., & Rossi, E. (1989). *Hypnotherapy: An exploratory casebook.* New York: Irvington.

Erickson, M., & Rossi, E. (1989). *The February man: Evolving consciousness and identity in hypnotherapy.* New York: Brunner/Mazel.

Erickson, M., Rossi, E., & Rossi, I. (1976). *Hypnotic realities.* New York: Irvington.

Lynn, S., Weekes, J., Matyi, C., & Neufeld, V. (1988). Direct versus indirect suggestions, archaic involvement, and hypnotic experience. *Journal of Abnormal Psychology, 97*(3), 296–301.

Rossi, E. (1986). *The psychobiology of mind-body: New concept in therapeutic hypnosis.* New York: Irvington.

Rossi, E., & Cheek, D. (1988). *Mind-body therapy: Ideodynamic healing in hypnosis.* New York: W. W. Norton.

Stone, J., & Lundy, R. (1985). Behavioral compliance with direct and indirect body movement suggestions. *Journal of Abnormal Psychology, 94*(3), 256–263.

Commentary

Stephen G. Gilligan, Ph.D.

Ernest Rossi began this hour-long presentation with a brief description of the fundamental ideas underlying his approach to psychotherapy. Because these ideas guide his subsequent demonstrations, they merit citation and commentary.

A first hypothesis set forth by Rossi is that creative moments involving an inner "ah-ha" are the essence of psychotherapy. In setting forth this idea, Rossi emphasizes the intrapersonal world as more important than the interpersonal in terms of therapeutic change. My own view is that both are equally important; the therapist using hypnosis needs to balance inner development with some equivalent outer expression. Otherwise, the client may feel better during the session but not act any differently between sessions, and the changes do not generalize to their relevant contexts. In this regard, Erickson's work demonstrated a balance between inner (hypnotic) processes and outer (strategic) expressions.

A second, related hypothesis is that creative moments can be stimulated by hypnosis, which Rossi sees as a subject-based inner process in which the role of the hypnotist is secondary. While Erickson promoted this view, which is a reaction to the dominant myth of hypnotist-dominant hypnosis, I don't think it accurately describes the work of either Rossi or Erickson. While Ericksonian hypnotherapy is based on the naturalistic experience of clients, it also relies on the skillful guidance and supervision of the therapist. This suggests an interpersonal model of hypnosis in which experience is co-constructed by the cooperative relationship between therapist and client (Gilligan, 1987). In this view, the important distinction is "mind-in-relationship," i.e., reconnecting the client's experiential life to larger contexts, both intrapersonally and interpersonally. *Relationship* is the key process by which this occurs and, thus, should be emphasized as the central aspect of the hypnotherapeutic work.

A third hypothesis is that trance is a naturalistic process best elicited via the client's ongoing experience rather than by standardized instructions or other artificial techniques. This idea is central to Ericksonian hypnotherapy, as it emphasizes the client's emotional experience as the basis for both trance induction and therapeutic change. Rossi's demonstrations beautifully illustrate how clients' dreams are one example of such naturalistic bases for technique. Other examples are symptoms, emotional memories, skills, childhood learnings, interpersonal relationships, and ongoing behaviors.

A fourth hypothesis is that hypnosis involves what Rossi calls the "language of facilitation." That is, the therapist elicits trance and guides change via various linguistic patterns. Rossi cites three of these patterns. The first are questions that bypass conscious involvement and access unconscious participation. In asking questions like "What part of your body feels most comfortable right now?", the hypnotherapist orients attention experientially inward, thereby stimulating therapeutic trance processes. A second linguistic pattern is what Rossi calls "channeling," which involves the principle of ideodynamicism. This principle, which is central to all forms of hypnosis, involves asking subjects to "allow their "unconscious" to "channel" or express ideas autonomously from their volitional control. Examples include "Let your hand begin to lift effortlessly" and "Let your unconscious mind begin to activate some emotional resource relevant to this problem." Encouraging this type of process is the essence of hypnosis.

A third linguistic pattern emphasized by Rossi is the "implied directive." This involves linking an inner hypnotic response with a hypnotic behavior, for example, "When your hand begins to lift up, that special dream will begin" or "You will go deeply into trance when your eyes close." This pattern allows subjects to proceed at their own rate, while providing the therapist with important ongoing feedback in terms of when the client is initiating or completing some suggested processes. The suggested hypnotic behaviors also provide subjects with subjectively compelling experiences of their own hypnotic involvement, thereby alleviating any doubts that might hamper the therapeutic explorations.

Gloria

Having presented his ideas, Rossi then works with his first volunteer. His technique is deceptively simple: He merely asks the subject to describe a meaningful dream. In doing so, he solicits a emotionally based experiential process as the basis for hypnotic explorations. As the subject elaborates her dream, Rossi relaxes and receives her verbal and nonverbal communications. It is as if he becomes the hypnotic subject for the moment, allowing the subject's presentation to touch and influence his unconscious processes.

As Rossi begins to focus nonverbally and to nod with the subject, she hypnotically responds by developing absorption and partial catalepsy. Rossi ratifies and deepens this initial response via verbal pacing of ongoing behavior, encouragement and nonverbal slowing down. When the woman responds to these naturalistic deepening techniques, Rossi encourages further trance development and then suggests unconscious exploration of the dream.

Interestingly, Rossi then immediately turns to the audience and describes the woman's processes in hypnotic terms. Shifting attention away from the subject provides "room" for her own explorations. The statements to the audience also constitute indirect suggestions to the subject. (In the clinical office, this could be done by talking with someone else, or by telling a story about someone else. Each technique shifts the spotlight of attention away from the subject while continuing to speak to his or her unconscious mind.)

After a while the woman reorients and briefly shares her experience. Rossi acknowledges her and then uses her natural post-trance hypnotic responsiveness to talk about ultradian rhythms. These comments also constitute indirect suggestions, in that post-trance consciousness is especially receptive to therapeutic suggestions.

As a clinical demonstration, the brevity of the work raises the question of how it might be applied in a therapy situation in relation to a presenting problem. One possibility is that such a piece of work might be interspersed within a session, such as when a client is at an impasse. Another possibility is that it could serve as part of a fractionation technique, wherein a series of successively deeper trances is initiated, with brief discussions sandwiched between them.

Another clinical issue concerns the connection of the trance experience to target areas of the client's life. This is where the strategic and tasking elements of Erickson's therapy were especially prominent. It seems that Rossi assumes that inner hypnotic work is sufficient for generating therapeutic changes. My own clinical experience suggests that it is not; usually, the therapist needs to make provisions for such generalizations to occur.

Sally

Rossi begins his second demonstration by again eliciting a dream report. The dream is long and complex, so Rossi sifts through it to identify meaningful entry points. The subject becomes emotional when talking about the "fear of reaching new places," whereupon Rossi begins experientially to focus her attention inward. This is another nice demonstration of using the subject's emotional arousal as the basis for trance development. Rossi orients the subject's attention to the spontaneous emotional quivering in her face, defines the experience as therapeutic ("It's trying to tell us something"), and then uses the experiential responses as the basis for trance development. He does this by using the simple hypnotic patterns of pacing and leading behavior, both verbally and nonverbally.

Rossi also uses his implied directives by suggesting that if her unconscious wants to receive "something," her eyes will close. This is an active yet subtle naturalistic use of the ideodynamic principle that is the basis for hypnosis. In this instance, it is used to receive ongoing information from the subject's unconscious mind regarding how to proceed. This is essential information for the hypnotist, and also provides the subject with "convincer" and deepening experiences.

Rossi builds on this response by suggesting that when the hand reaches the lap, a meaningful experience will occur. This implied directive nicely demonstrates the Ericksonian techniques of building on small responses, subject-paced processes, and receiving ongoing feedback from the subject.

When the subject reorients, she notes how her ideodynamic response was automatic and *seemed to be initiated nonverbally*, before Rossi said anything. This comment reflects the importance of nonverbal communication between hypnotist and subject. Like any intensely experiential relationship, much of hypnosis consists of a *nonverbal* conversation based on minimal, mutually influencing cues. This circular model suggests that the hypnotherapist can best operate as an experiential participant-observer.

When the subject describes feeling the repetitive message in trance of "It's time to take that climb," Rossi verbally and nonverbally acknowledges her while also nonverbally (via a deep sigh) suggesting that she can "let go" as she does so. On this note, the demonstration ends.

Again, one is left wondering how Rossi would proceed in a clinical context at this point. Would he end here, or would he offer further therapeutic suggestions, either indirectly (e.g., through stories) or directly (e.g., by presenting tasks)? The question, of course, is how to make the hypnosis therapeutic by ensuring that there are bridges from the hypnotic experiences to the target contexts. The danger in giving no bridges is that the hypnotic experience, while impressive, doesn't make a real difference in the client's life. The dangers in being too directive include eliciting defense mechanisms, providing wrong directions, and having the changes felt as therapist initiated. Thus, it seems that a therapist must find a balance point for each client.

Fay

Rossi begins with his third subject by taking a few deep breaths. This simple act is a nice reminder of the importance of the therapist tuning into his or her own nonverbal processes as a basis for unconscious creativity.

As the subject describes the "pink light" featured in the dream, Rossi and the audience laugh. When he discovers that it isn't funny for the client, he apologizes simply. This is a important demonstration of the need for the therapist to acknowledge mistakes. Rossi then "resets" by again taking several deep breaths, thereby showing one example of how the therapist can meet the important demand of having some simple "centering" techniques available.

After probing for emotionally relevant aspects of the dream, Rossi feeds them back ("spiritual," "feminine," "pink light in sky"). This absorbs attention and elicits a therapeutic trance. Rossi then ratifies and frames the behavioral response of eye shifting as indicative of trance then turns to the audience to suggest (to them directly and the subject indirectly) that she is shifting to a "slightly deeper level" of work where her "whole system [is] relaxed now as she focuses on the inner work." He then pauses to allow the subject to respond to this indirect suggestion.

His continued use of the phrase, "that's it," shows the value of letting subjects know that you are in touch with them. It is important that the hypnotist notice and support hypnotic responses. This simple ratification not only assures the subject, it allows the hypnotist to develop a rhythmic and repetitive hypnotic presentation.

As the subject responds with hypnotic deepening, Rossi suggests dissociation from emotion. This timely suggestion utilizes the hypnotic ability to be "apart from and a part of" experience to encourage a deep connection with, yet appropriate distance from, an emotional memory. As the client manifests an emotional response, Rossi ratifies and softly supports it, then suggests that the tears bear a therapeutic message. He then guides her to receive the message, let go, and experience an integration. In doing so, he demonstrates that it is not essential that the therapist always know the content of the client's hypnotic experience; the therapist need only provide the proper guidance and support. This involves nonverbal centering, support and assurance.

Given that the process accessed by the subject seems to be a deeply emotional one, Rossi recognizes that it need not (and probably should not) be integrated fully within the short session. He thus offers posthypnotic suggestions for continued integration in nocturnal dreams. In doing so, Rossi demonstrates the important idea that most therapeutic work is only begun, not finished, within the formal trance. Post-trance opportunities for integration of hypnotic learnings are essential in hypnotherapy. Thus, the suggestion for nocturnal dream integrations is a nice technique that can be helpful for many clients.

The client reorients and feels vulnerable. This is quite common when emotional trance work has occurred. The therapist needs to recognize and respect this, for example, by not moving into "interrogation" or analysis of the experience. It is helpful to remember that the unconscious is active and. vulnerable before and after formal trance work.

As the client describes her experience in terms of letting go of fear, she presents her vulnerability. Rossi meets the client by sharing some of his own vulnerability, thereby offering an exceptional model of the therapist being willing and able to operate at the same level of experiential involvement as the client. His sharing of himself takes the "spotlight" off the client and provides greater "room" for her feelings to be presented and consolidated.

Janet

The fourth and final demonstration subject relates an emotionally intense dream in which she was moving toward "infinity," then had to return because it was "not the time." Apparently sensitive to this, Rossi does not use the dream to develop trance. Instead, he first orients attention to the similarity of his eyes and her eyes (shifting attention), then introduces the simple induction technique of an ideomotoric "magnetic pull" of the hands. As the subject develops this hypnotic response, Rossi suggests that she only momentarily dip back into the "infinity" dream, make a "fast grab" at something, and then quickly reorient back from trance. These suggestions parallel the style reflected in the subject's dream descriptions, thereby supporting and utilizing it.

Though the subject was in trance for only a brief time, she reoriented with amnesia. While Rossi acknowledges this as evidence of a deep trance, he refuses her request to repeat what was said during trance. He emphasizes the importance of protecting and supporting any amnesias developed by the subject's unconscious, thereby demonstrating in yet another way his respect for the client's individual style of responding.

Summary

Rossi's work with the four demonstration subjects provides an excellent illustration of how Ericksonian hypnotic processes can be used in a simple yet sophisticated way. Rossi's work is almost entirely based on using the subject's experiential processes as the vehicle for hypnotic induction and therapeutic exploration. Rossi shows how the therapist can proceed by tuning into himself or herself, connecting nonverbally, and receiving and amplifying hypnotic communications from the subject. His trust and support of the client's integrity is evident throughout his work as is his genuine caring and sensitivity.

Equally impressive is his use of naturalistic techniques of Ericksonian hypnosis. In addition to his three cited techniques of accessing questions, "channeling" suggestions, and implied directives, Rossi also consistently uses techniques of ratifying and framing responses, nonverbal and verbal pacing and leading, building on small responses, using emotionally relevant symbols as the basis for induction and utilization, pretrance and post-trance hypnotic suggestions, nonverbal suggestion, posthypnotic suggestion, and nonverbal centering.

It is especially refreshing to note that Rossi applies these techniques in a way quite distinct from Erickson. In doing so, he encourages each therapist to find his or her own way of communicating hypnotically in a therapeutic fashion.

Reference

Gilligan, S. G. (1987). *Therapeutic trances: The cooperation principle in Ericksonian hypnotherapy.* New York: Brunner/Mazel.

Using Metaphor and the Interspersal Technique

Jeffrey K. Zeig, Ph.D.

The patient volunteered from the audience and mentioned her problem. When she came up to the stage, she was asked to repeat her concern.

Zeig: What have you been troubled with . . .

Silvia: Hm-hm.

Zeig: . . . and can you repeat the situation and what you want to accomplish?

Silvia: Well, I think basically over the last couple of months my denial is not as great as it used to be. And I fear that we don't have a whole lot of time left as a planet because of the nuclear race and the threat that we are all under. And it is fine until, usually, when I am getting into the car to go to work. And it is at that time that I wonder, why am I bothering to go to work? When I have to say good-bye I don't have time for this. Hm. And it becomes quite distressing because when I get to work I have to try to forget about it and to start doing my work again.

Zeig: So really what you want to accomplish is to bolster up your denial so that you can push the real threat that is there into the background and be able to enjoy the tasks that you have in front of you. You don't want to forget about it?

Silvia: I feel the denial is very frightening to me . . .

Zeig: Yes, hm-hm.

Silvia: . . . as well because if we continue to deny the threat that we are under we're not going to do anything about it.

Zeig: Right.

Silvia: So perhaps it's a feeling of helplessness.

Zeig: Perhaps you can change that to "repress." So just to push into the

---

Transcript of a demonstration given in Los Angeles, December 1984.

background the threat, but not deny it and block it out. You just want to have it in the background when you need it in the background so that it doesn't trouble you.

Silvia: Right.

Zeig: But you want to know it's there, so that there are things . . . because there are things you might want to do about it. Right?

Silvia: Yes.

Zeig: All right, what have you done to try to repress things more?

Silvia: I really don't know. I don't know what I do to repress things. I guess I try to feel each moment's importance—this moment with this individual—that this client is going to be important, too. And we have to keep going. And that sometimes works.

Zeig: So it's like you give yourself a little pep talk?

Silvia: Right.

Zeig: And then, say you wanted to make it worse. You got this crazy idea in your mind that you really wanted to plague yourself with the threat. How would you do that?

Silvia: That's not very hard to do.

Zeig: Hm-hm.

Silvia: I just read the paper. *(laughter)* I listen to the news. I mean at times I won't listen to the news. I just go to bed before it comes on because I am tempted to sit and watch it, but I don't want to because it just sort of undoes what I just finished doing for myself.

Zeig: Right. And then this experience of trance. How do you experience hypnosis? What's it like for you?

Silvia: Actually, it's a feeling of purple and red.

Zeig: Aha, aha, hm . . .

Silvia: And a kind of going down with purples and reds.

Zeig: And the purple and reds are round you? A part of you?

Silvia: A part of me, more inside.

Zeig: Hm-hm. And as you begin to remember . . . that feeling, the pleasant feeling of going down . . . and the purples and the reds . . . you begin to slow yourself down.

Silvia: Hm-hm.

Zeig: And you can perhaps begin to get some of those physical sensations . . . that go along.

Silvia: Hm.

Zeig: And then you can recognize that you can begin *to look forward* . . . to that point . . . in which you can *just close your eyes* . . . so *(she closes her eyes)* that you can . . . really transport . . . yourself . . . along that path . . . so that you can, Silvia, really become yourself . . . even more . . . absorbed . . . even more . . . with those developing sensations of comfort. And, Silvia, as you take part . . . in that process . . . you can realize that your *neck muscles* . . . have begun to make an accommodation . . . so that you can *find yourself* . . . *straight ahead* . . . *(she moves her head slightly) again* even more . . . yourself . . . absorbed in the experiencing. There is something rather charming about that. Something charming . . . and disarming . . . because it also allows you . . . this moment . . . *to turn your ear more toward me (she moves her head)* . . . so that you can hear . . . even more clearly, and it is really charming and disarming, and . . . you can recognize . . . that when I direct my voice towards you, I'll speak to you. And you can use this time . . . to just follow down . . . that path of color.

(To audience) Now in working with Silvia, there are certain things that I wanted to find out: I wanted to get a concrete description of the problem. I also wanted to get an understanding of what she has done to solve the problem because then I'd know not to try those things. I also wanted to know what she could do to make the problem worse, because that helps me in planning out my strategy. Perhaps I could even use that for symptom prescription or for creating some kind of a bind. But then, as I started the hypnosis with Silvia, I wanted to build the responsiveness, because really the essence of hypnosis is gaining the patient's cooperation and gaining the responsiveness of the patient. And I wanted to learn something about Silvia's responses to minimal cues, and I learned that Silvia is really attentive to minimal cues. Not only is she attentive to minimal cues, she is responsive. And so once I have that kind of responsiveness, then I know I have rapport. I know that there is a sense of trust in the situation, and I also know from Silvia's description that she is motivated to do something about this problem because it's really been plaguing her. There is no therapy that's going to happen without trust, no therapy that's going to happen without a sense of empathy. "This is a difficult situation you and I are involved in and I am here and available to help you." And so it's at *that* point, when I see this responsiveness to minimal cues, when I *know* that there is some cooperation, that I can feel "Yes, I've got the nod from the patient, the go-ahead from the patient to be able to proceed with the utilization."

And, Silvia, you are comfortable, *(she nods her head)* are you not? You are comfortable. *(she nods her head)* And, Silvia, you can understand . . . that your head nod . . . is different. It's not the ordinary *(she nods her head)* kind of head nod. It's more the unconscious *(she nods her head)* variety. And Silvia shows that very nice perseveration . . . of the nod. And sometimes that perseveration can go on for quite a long time . . . and, Silvia, *(she smiles)* where are you now?

Silvia: Smiling, because I realized my head was still moving.

Zeig: Yes. Smiling, because you realize that your head was still moving. And it's nice to really know that your head *can* move. It's nice to really understand . . . that your head *now* is in a different . . . position . . . than it was before. And your voice may have sounded a bit differently—to you. And the translation from thoughts into words, that could be a little bit different. And there is a certain immediate sense of comfort. Can you describe that?

Silvia: A sort of red. *(she smiles)*

Zeig: A red. And any blue in there?

Silvia: The blue and red makes purple. *(she smiles)*

Zeig: And the blue and red makes the purple. And that experience . . . of being sort of a bodiless mind . . . just absorbed in that purple, and just letting the . . . purple . . . transpose itself . . . on to your immediate experience . . . and letting that purple . . . transposition that you have . . . take you even more into that charming and pleasant state . . . of being yourself . . . absorbed. And Silvia, certainly you can attend to me, and you can listen, and you can respond. And insofar as you are concerned, is there anyone else here? *(she shakes head)* There is nobody else here. And that experience . . . of the people somehow fading . . . into the background. It's really a rather pleasant experience and it allows you to attend . . . to what's really *(she nods)* important . . . because, Silvia, you can understand that the experience of hypnosis . . . it can be almost like drifting off . . . into a colorful dream, and what's here . . . is important . . . and what's there . . . somehow just fades. But physically you could recognize . . . even more . . . that really anytime that you wanted to make any of those small adjustments to maximize you own sense of comfort . . . and well-being . . . you could feel free to do that. For example, to go inside . . . even more . . . you could just keep your eyes closed, look up to the top of your head, *(she takes a deep breath)* take a deep breath, and notice how that helps you . . . to let yourself get down . . . even more . . . into that state of being immediately absorbed . . . in the experience . . . and in the dream.

Perhaps you could dream . . . about a village . . . in the middle . . . of an overgrown forest . . . and the village is a village that's . . . being . . . surrounded by not only an overgrown forest but by horrible dragons. Very, very real dragons, fire-breathing dragons. Now inside the village . . . the villagers create . . . huge defenses to keep the dragons out—to keep the dragons at bay. Very thick defenses. Unfortunately, at times, the defenses seem to break, and the roar of the dragons rings in people's ears. Sometimes, the hot breath of the dragon can be felt . . . by the poor villagers. Now the villagers have tried . . .

to do things about the dragon. They've bolstered their defenses. They've sent their young people . . . to fight the dragon. They have organized groups of young people . . . to go out against the dragons. But each time, the young people have come back defeated, yet more resolved: "We are going to do something . . . about those horrible dragons." Yet, some people in the village have become increasingly alarmed . . . about the horrible dragons. And they . . . think, time and time again, "Those dragons . . . are overwhelming. We must do something about them." And yet, bolstering up the defenses does not seem to work. As a matter of fact, the defenses have even been isolating . . . because they have prevented commerce and interchange . . . with other villages. And some of the people have lived in despair. And so it seems like a horrible situation—an overwhelming situation.

Now in the center . . . of the village, there lived a very dedicated young woman. . . . And she decided, "Something needs to be done . . . about the situation. I need to do something . . . about the situation today." And so she went out . . . on a . . . quest. But then she got . . . intimidated. She thought to herself, "This is overwhelming. It's ridiculous. Nothing can be done about the dragons. They just pervade that forest." But then she thought, "Perhaps I can visit . . . the wizard. Perhaps I can talk with the wizard. Perhaps he can give me some advice . . . that I can use . . . in (she takes a deep breath) dealing with the dragons."

The wizard said, "Sit down . . . in my easy chair . . . and immediately feel yourself . . . at home . . . in my easy chair. Now I would like you to recognize . . . that there are . . . so many different kinds of tears. There are tears of anger (she is crying); there are tears of rage; there are tears of frustration; there are tears of fear; there are tears of confusion; tears of denial; tears of joy; tears of relief. And there are tears that wash away . . . some old hurts . . . so that they can fade . . . with those drying tears."

The wizard said, "Just sit in the easy chair . . . and spend a few moments (she swallows) looking into the flames . . . in the fire." The wizard said, "When you look into the flames . . . they are really colorful. And just like, as a child, you could look into the clouds, and see faces and spaces and places, so you can look into the flames, and see faces and spaces and places. It's really charming to do. And when the flames are totally consumed, then you can . . . just close your eyes and drift off . . . and really immediately listen to me . . . even more clearly . . . understanding that you are certainly far enough away from the heat . . . that none of the heat needs to get to you. But the warmth . . . can certainly be there. It can certainly be there appreciably."

(To audience) Now, one of the steps of the process of hypnotherapy is to get responsiveness, because if there is no responsiveness, there is no therapy. And once you have the responsiveness, then you need to be able to show an empathy for the situation, and you need to reflect back to the person that you empathically understand what the problem is. And you don't need to empathize with the situation in this Rogerian sense—"I understand that you have concerns, I understand that you are upset"—but you can also empathize with the situation indirectly. You can empathize with the situation metaphorically. And I think that empathizing with the situation metaphorically allows you to reach the person on much more profound levels.

The essence of this indirection is to be just one step removed from the situation. So you know what the situation is. And then you can express it one step removed. As you express it one step removed, it allows the person to energize the situation. And, it's really the person who has the power to change and create some of the new possibilities. So then once you start, and once you've completed empathizing with the situation, and once you've laid some of the groundwork for the therapy, then you can begin to re-create and re-access some of the resources that the person has for dealing with these situations.

(Silvia nods) And, Silvia, in the dream . . . the wizard says: "Just close your eyes, look up, take an easy breath, and let yourself really drift down . . . inside . . . because as you drift inside . . . you may reflect . . . on certain colors . . . that can really transpose themselves . . . into the situation. And you may even catch a glimpse . . . of a memory . . . of how pleasant . . . those sensations, those developing sensations can be."

The wizard said, "Now, although you probably are not attending to it . . . now, you may have noticed . . . that near the fire . . . there is a pressure cooker. It's a really old pressure cooker. It's very special. Now the way that pressure cooker works is that you put the meat, and the potatoes, and the vegetables inside. And you put some of the water inside, really important that you have the water. And then you start *to apply heat* . . . from the outside, and you use that heat . . . to build up steam, and *you need the steam* . . . *to get things cooking.* And the steam builds up pressure, and you *really need the pressure* . . . *to get things cooking.* But you also realize . . . that you have the gasket and the seal. And, also you have the valve on top, and you adjust the valve so that you have 5 pounds of pressure, 10 pounds of pressure, or 15 pounds of pressure inside, because remember that you really need the pressure . . . to get things cooking.

"And there is really *a certain security* . . . in seeing the valve . . . *nodding* up and down, because then you know that the pressure *is right inside*. And sometimes you see condensation of moisture on the outside, and that lets you know that things are right. And you hear the sound . . . of the pressure cooker. And the sound lets you know . . . that things are really working right. Now there is some care that you need to take. You need to make sure that the valve is *working properly* . . . so that you can have the right amount of pressure. You don't need to attend to the pressure cooker once it is working, because you know that your unconscious mind will attend to the condensation, attend to the nodding of the valve up and down, attend to the sound. And you can just let your unconscious mind attend to that sound. Just like when you have a baby and the baby is asleep in the room. The mother is able to listen . . . to the baby, and even in a deep sleep, if the baby cries, the mother will hear it, because her activating system . . . is there and her activating system is really tuned in, but she can still let herself enjoy the sleep."

And, Silvia, you understand . . . that in a dream, things fade, and yet there's an orientation. And you are orientated in the room. And you are orientated to the bed, even though your mind can be certainly somewhere else—involved in the colors, involved in the immediate experience, in the dream.

And so the wizard said, "Now, that pressure cooker, it *needs* to be used. You would not want to just keep it on the shelf. You'd really want to make sure . . . that it's clear, and that the valves are in good shape, and that the gaskets are really working right, and that the seals are there. And, as a matter of fact, *you need the heat*, because it is the heat that's used to build up steam. And you need the steam, because it is the steam that gets things cooking."

And the wizard said, "There are other things . . . to really understand. That you *can* . . . recognize and that you *can* . . . even realize, in a straightforward way, that you can take straight ahead *(she moves her head)* of yourself." The wizard said, "You might want to imagine yourself . . . going down . . . into a very special place, sort of a room of your own, sitting yourself down in an easy chair, and again feeling yourself at home in an easy chair . . . recognizing . . . that you could drift off . . . into a trance . . . and that you could experience . . . that balance . . . as a certain kind . . . of relaxation, the kind of relaxation . . . that you've had . . . many, many times . . . in the past. The kind of relaxation . . . that you can have . . . many, many times . . . in the future. The kind of relaxation . . . that you can have . . . in tense moments, because in tense moments . . . do you want to be . . . looking around . . . in this way, or that? Or experience yourself hidden in this way, or that? Or would you rather just look up, and take an easy breath, and allow yourself to just fade . . . into that pleasant state . . . of really . . . colorful comfort."

And as you looked around, and as you look out the window of the room, you might remember from time to time . . . that things could seem . . . awfully . . . different. As a matter of fact you could notice that there were . . . colors, that there were flashes of red. But any time that you wanted to, you could just, in a straightforward way, recognize . . . that you *could* . . . just add . . . some of that pleasant blue . . . and give yourself the go-ahead . . . to develop some of those sensations . . . of enduring comfort . . .

Now another thing about that room . . . is that, in a moment, something special, another you, could walk into that room, a you that really represented . . . the best you . . . that was inside. And can you see that . . . other you standing there now straight and tall? And can you recognize that that you . . . is more solid *(she nods)* than transparent? And yet there may be a transparent quality about it, too, which would be okay. And could you also attend . . . to the fact that, somehow, it seems important to note . . . that there is a certain orientation, one in which the point in the middle of the forehead . . . is lined-up . . . with the point in the middle of the lips, which is lined-up . . . with the point in the middle of the forehead? *(pause)* Now, in a moment, something unusual . . . that can be done . . . which is that you can . . . put yourself . . . inside . . . that more ideal you, so that you can see . . . what it looks like . . . out of her eyes, and so that you can get the sensation of what it's like . . . to have that point in the middle of your forehead, aligned with the point of the middle of your lips, aligned with the point of the middle of your breast-bone, so that you can take some time . . . to memorize . . . that sensation . . . carefully, so that it *can (she nods her head)* become a part . . . of your immediate experience, and something else strange to notice . . . is that there might be a penchant, a real immediate penchant, to attend to those flashes of purple . . . that are apparent . . . to you. And when you've really accomplished that, you could *indicate* . . . and . . . really *go ahead* . . . even more . . .

"Yes," the wizard said, "Now, there may not be anything that can be done, really, about those dragons now. But I want you to take that energy—really organized—so that you *can go straight ahead . . . and really continue . . . that process.* You know those dragons are awfully difficult, and they really are there, and they really need to be pushed back. It will take quite a long time, maybe even more time than you have. But you *go out on that quest,* and *you use that time . . . constructively,* and then you can *remember, from time to time,* some of the things that we have discussed."

And in the dream, the dream can fade ٧ . . . into the background, because, Silvia, you have had the experience . . . of arousing yourself . . . from a dream not being able to fully remember . . . the dream. And yet the feelings, the comfortable feelings from the dream, may be there, down *inside* you, immediately recognizable. Almost sometimes, like, when you have heard a tune . . . that you enjoy, and you are whistling that particular tune . . . to yourself from time to time, and you are hearing it, and you are using it as background. That feeling can be there. And so, just going inside, and just really . . . taking in . . . more of that immediate sensation, you can . . . begin to bring back . . . yourself . . . reorientation . . . recognizing that you can make the reorientations . . . straight ahead . . . at your own pace. Perhaps taking an easy breath and rousing yourself . . . fully alert and wide awake . . . all over . . . reorienting . . . in the right way . . . for you. *(long pause)* Hi! *(she takes a deep breath, wipes her eyes, rubs her hands)*

Silvia: Hi.

Zeig: What can you say about the experience?

Silvia: It is certainly not warm up here.

Zeig: Not warm. Cold hands?

Silvia: Cold hands.

Zeig: Yeah, mine, too.

Silvia: And you knew it wouldn't be warm near the fire. *(both laugh)*

Zeig: And what was most compelling about it? I would normally not do this, I wouldn't ask you. But because this is somewhat of a teaching situation, I think that we could learn something.

Silvia: Well, being in my own home, watching myself walk through the front door, which is actually also the door of the room of my private office, so actually I was sitting in my office, which is also my living room, and watching myself walk through the door.

Zeig: Watching yourself walk through the door.

Silvia: And um . . . and you said something about orientation, something about foreheads, and right at that point I was face to face with a picture of my mother when she was 16, and um, that felt real significant to me—that when I walked in my room I walked there.

Zeig: She is an active person?

Silvia: She is dead.

Zeig: She was an active person? Yes? A political person?

Silvia: No.

Zeig: Hm.

Silvia: But active, yes, she had five kids.

Zeig: Yes.

(Laughter)

Zeig: You can't know what people will be doing with their imagery so, it's interesting to learn afterward about the person's associational processes, certainly when you are doing ongoing therapy it's helpful to know something about the associational processes.

   Well, there's time for one or two brief questions.

Zeig: The question relates to the references to "straightforward posture." Right. Well, our behavior affects our feelings as much as our feelings affect our behavior. And sometimes, when you want to create an anchor, a possibility of an anchor for a person, then you might want to use some physical cues so that the person can cue themselves into certain states. And it's the seeding, I think, that's most important—that you don't just give an anchor to a person, but that if you have the idea that it might be possible to use this, then you start very early in the process to establish those cues.

Silvia: That sets off something new, well I think it could have been, when using those words of yours, my neck muscle hurt. A lot in here. I remember being conscious of how that was aching. And now it's fine.

Zeig: It's fine.

Silvia: So I don't know . . .

Zeig: Well, okay.

Member of the audience: I think I noticed a difference in your voice. Afterwards it sounded more, I guess, centered, clearer.

Zeig: There is more resonance in Silvia's voice.

Silvia: When I am nervous, I have a higher pitch.

Zeig: Yeah.

Silvia: So, perhaps, when I started my voice had a higher pitch. Because when I get more relaxed, and I feel a lot more relaxed now than I did before, mm, so perhaps that's what it was an indication of.

Zeig: Okay. We need to stop.

Commentary

Jeffrey K. Zeig, Ph.D.

The patient for this demonstration was a female physician who was attending the 1984 Erickson Foundation Seminar. While she was seated in the audience, I talked to her before agreeing to work with her in order to ensure that her problem could be addressed in this particular setting. This would be a complete therapy, and there would be no chance for a follow-up session.

She said she experienced anxiety about nuclear disaster. My therapy goals, therefore, were to help her locate her own resources for action—action which could reduce her sense of powerlessness.

The goals for a demonstration differ from psychotherapy, and my demonstrations only resemble the therapy I conduct in my private office. One difference is the fact that I am not merely concerned with the patient, but also with offering a method professionals can use in clinical practice. The teaching goals can interfere with the therapy goals, and the quality of the relationship in a demonstration is different from the relationship in clinical practice.

In this session, I told a metaphor about a dragon. I rarely invent stories for patients, preferring to relate real stories, which convey more feeling of immediacy. However, I use some made-up stories in my clinical practice, and, in this case, I decided the invented metaphor would make a valuable demonstration for the audience and also serve as a useful vehicle for the patient.

Analyzing a therapy is a bit like analyzing a poem. If one treats it rationally, some of the integrity is lost. I will mention some of the techniques that were most important to me as I worked with the patient.

I offered suggestions during each phase of contact: diagnostic, induction, and treatment. In the diagnostic period, my initial suggestions were an attempt to "dislodge" the problem. While the patient initially talked about "denial," I tried to substitute the idea of "repression," because it was one step less than denial. My rationale for this substitution was that if I could elicit one change in the problem, I could elicit others.

If I had to do it over again, I would have gotten more diagnostic information, including how specifically "denial" got in her way. But, I thought I had enough information to begin, so I offered a conversational induction using her concepts of "purple and red" and "going down." I could not fully know what those concepts meant to her, but they were important aspects of *her* experiential language, so I used them.

During the induction, I presented embedded suggestions in the form of minimal cures, such as *"Look forward,"* "Find yourself *straight ahead,"* *"Turn your head toward me,"* until I could see that she was demonstrably responsive. I took her responses to indicate the induction period was over, and that utilization could begin. By virtue of her response to my indirect suggestions, I concluded that rapport, trust, and openness to suggestion existed, and resistance was minimal. Also, I returned to the idea of head posture a number of times in the course of treatment.

As I proceeded to the end of the induction, I introduced the concept "charming and disarming." Because of her concern about nuclear threat, the word "disarming" could have special meaning: I wanted to desensitize any excess emotion by presenting the idea of disarming in a purely positive way. I returned to this concept again, eventually offering the word "charming" in a way that she, herself, could associate to "disarming."

After talking to the audience, I ratified the trance by noting her perseverative nodding. I took this head movement to have symbolic meaning: She was saying "yes" to me. I build on her orientation to her head by offering positive symbolic suggestions that her "head could be in a different place"—that therapeutic change was already occurring.

When Silvia responded to my subsequent suggestions that "voices fade," I trusted that she could generalize this skill. I assumed that she had her problem in mind by virtue of asking for help. Hence, she could apply any technique from the hypnosis to her problem; that is, she could transfer the fading of voices to the fading (repression) of her concerns. She was accessing a mechanism that could be used as a concrete solution. When she later started crying, I returned to the idea of fading as a way to control unruly emotion. Further, I offered the idea that one can take something positive out of an uncomfortable background when I presented the concept of taking the "warmth" out of the flames while minimizing the heat. I knew she would have life experience of taking positive things out of an uncomfortable foreground, and I offered the possibility that she could bring that skill into the present situation. If she could bring it into the immediate therapy, she could apply it in the future, especially in relationship to the problem.

Throughout the session, the colors were a resource. If she could bring the purple haze of the trance into the situation of her thoughts of nuclear threat, perhaps that would help accomplish her goals. The idea of utilizing both the color and the fading were brought into the therapy and tied to action—that of taking a deep breath. With this addition, there were cognitive, emotional and behavioral things she could *do* if she felt overwhelmed.

Later in the session I provided suggestions within a "pressure cooker" metaphor. I offered a behavioral cue of "putting her head on straight" (the three aligned points). This was another behavioral tool she could use when the feelings became too great. The alignment of the head was seeded (see Zeig, in press, for further information on seeding) early in the induction. Earlier references to her head posture and her head "being in a different place" would now have new meaning.

There was something I missed during the reorientation period: During trance I talked with the patient about the positive interject she could create during the time that she was in the "room of her own" and I emphasized the transparent (trance-parent) quality of the figure. When she reoriented from the trance, she described a picture of her mother! At the time I did not realize how literally she was responding.

If I had to do it over again, there are three things I would change: 1) At the end of the session, I might have used a fantasy rehearsal technique, whereby the patient could orient to the future and practice using the tools garnered during the therapy to ameliorate the presenting problem. 2) I would have used a more interactive trance. Rather than speaking to a passive patient as I did, I would have had a discussion with her during hypnosis to secure more specific feedback. 3) I am not sure it was necessary to use so many techniques. Since Silvia was responsive and motivated, I may have been able to accomplish equally positive results with less work.

The effect of the therapy was positive. I saw Silvia at later meetings, and she reported that she accomplished her goal.

References

Zeig, J. K. (in press). Seeding. In J. Zeig & S. Gilligan (Eds.), *Brief therapy: Myths, methods and metaphors*. New York: Brunner/Mazel.

Commentary

William Hudson O'Hanlon, M.S.

Jeff Zeig starts this session with an intervention, skillfully using the assessment process as an intervention. More specifically, he uses the past tense when asking his client about her presenting complaint. He speaks to her, in almost the first sentence, about a problem "that you *have been* troubled with." In a paper presented at the First International Erickson Congress (1982), Zeig talks about the use of this linguistic method to promote the expectation of change. It's one of the common legacies that Jeff and I have from Erickson—deliberately using the assessment process as an intervention process from the first moments.

Before too long, still during the first few minutes of assessment, Zeig begins the use of the interspersal method of indirect suggestion that he intends to demonstrate in this session. In reflecting to the client, he tells her, "So, what you really want to do is to bolster your denial and *enjoy the tasks you have in front of you*." The italicized portion of the sentence is delivered in a different voice tone and volume and it constitutes the interspersed suggestion.

The session proceeds, and after a few minutes dialogue about the problem and previous attempted solutions (obviously drawing on the work of the MRI Brief Therapy Group, see Watzlawick et al., 1974) Zeig proceeds with more interspersed suggestions. This time the suggestions are a mixture of induction and treatment suggestions, again showing how Ericksonian approaches do not always make clear distinctions between the assessment/diagnosis, induction and treatment phases of therapy. His interspersed phrases include: *look forward; close your eyes; tran*sport; *Silvia, really become . . . even more absorbed; sense of trust; do something about this problem; comfort and well-being;* and *trust.*

Zeig eases into the induction by asking Silvia about previous trance experiences. She tells him that she has previously had a "feeling of purple and reds" as she enters trance. He indirectly suggests that she reevoke that experience by using verb tense as an indirect suggestion again. He asks her, "*Are* the purples and reds around you?" and "As you *begin to remember. . ."* This induction is classic conversational induction. The client is given no obvious signal that the trance induction is beginning. She just finds herself already in the experience without much thought (or chance to resist).

After induction, Silvia is offered two metaphors, a story about a village that is surrounded by a horrible dragon and an analogy about a pressure cooker. These metaphors seem to follow the Lanktons' multiple embedded metaphor model (Lankton & Lankton, 1983). The first story clearly matches Silvia's presenting concern and gives a model for solving that concern (the "matching metaphor"). A "dedicated young woman" decides "something needs to be done" and "I need to do something." She goes on a quest, where she encounters a wizard who tells her things that lead to the second metaphor about the pressure cooker. This seems to be the "resource metaphor," in which pressure is reframed as necessary to "get things cooking." The image of a "relief valve" is offered as an additional resource. More interspersed suggestions follow: *"relaxation . . . in the future . . . in tense moments . . . colorful comfort . . . go ahead."* These suggestions are linked to Silvia sitting in a comfortable chair in her house to ensure the transfer of the evoked resources to her everyday life.

Throughout the trance, Zeig seems attuned to Silvia's physical ————— in comments about her body movements and —————— in the story about

Zeig, J. (1982). Ericksonian approaches to promote abstinence from cigarette smoking. In J. Zeig (Ed.), *Ericksonian approaches to hypnosis and psychotherapy.* New York: Brunner/Mazel.

Weakland, J. & Fisch, R. (1974). *Change: Principles of problem formations and problem resolution.* New York: Norton.

what her unconscious or Zeig (either one or both are the wizard) has for her to solve her problem" It seemed like "doing a technique on a patient" to me. I much prefer genuine anecdotes that derive from the therapist's experience. There was an artificial feeling to much of the first part of the session, which seemed to dissolve as Zeig got more absorbed into trance and came across as more genuine. Along those lines, my favorite moment early in the session came after Zeig had asked Silvia what she could do to make her fear worse. She replied that all she had to do was to read the paper or watch TV. Zeig laughed and seemed genuinely "there" for a moment, not just a therapist doing a demonstration with a patient, but a human being in a human encounter with another.

Just one last point of difference. When Zeig suggests to Silvia that what she wants to do is to learn to repress better, I thought it a misstep. First, it seemed to dismiss her fears as groundless, implying that all she would have to do to resolve them was to repress them. She objected and told him that she didn't want to deny the nuclear threat. He quickly adjusted and rephrased her goal as wanting to push the threat into the background. I would have made a different distinction. I would have suggested that her fear was crippling and limiting her ability to do all she could to help rid the world of this threat, because she became paralyzed with discourage-ment. What I would have offered to help her do was to face the reality of it and let that strengthen her resolve to take effective action about the situation. Ultimately, I think that's where Zeig was heading in his treatment, as he interspersed suggestions about doing something several times during the demonstration, but I think he could have "paced" her conscious frame of reference more skillfully and respectfully.

Ultimately, my niggling differences aside, the proof of the pudding is in the eating. Silvia seemed to enjoy and obtain relief from the meal that was cooked up for her by Zeig in the pressure cooker of a workshop demonstration.

References

Lankton, S. & Lankton, C. (1983). *The answer within: A clinical framework of Ericksonian hypnotherapy.* New York: Brunner/M……